The "Feeling Great!" Wellness Program for Older Adults

ABOUT THE AUTHOR

Jules C. Weiss, MA, ATR, has been working as a counselor, art therapist, and in various health-related positions with older adults for over fifteen years. Mr. Weiss is trained by the YMCA as an exercise instructor and in other fitness specializations. He is the author of *Expressive Therapy With Elders and the Disabled* and numerous other publications about older adults.

Mr. Weiss was the Director of the "Feeling Great!" program at the Lee Circle YMCA in New Orleans, Louisiana. Currently, he is the Director of the Art Therapy Program at Salem College in Salem, West Virginia. Mr. Weiss is also a counselor and art therapist in private practice, a lecturer at colleges and conferences, and a consultant at various facilities.

The "Feeling Great!" Wellness Program for Older Adults

Jules C. Weiss

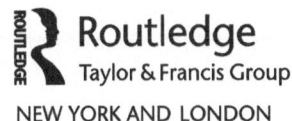
Routledge
Taylor & Francis Group

NEW YORK AND LONDON

The "Feeling Great!" Wellness Program for Older Adults has also been published as *Activities, Adaptation & Aging*, Volume 12, Numbers 3/4 1988.

First published 1988 by The Haworth Press, Inc.

Published 2014 by Routledge
605 Third Avenue, New York, NY 10017
4 Park Square, Milton Park, Abingdon, Oxon OX14 4RN

Routledge is an imprint of the Taylor & Francis Group, an informa business

LIBRARY OF CONGRESS
Library of Congress Cataloging-in-Publication Data

Weiss, Jules C.
    The "Feeling great!" wellness program for older adults / Jules C. Weiss.
        p.   cm.
    Also published as Activities, adaptation & aging, vol. 12, no. 3-4, 1988.
    Bibliography: p.
    Includes index.
    ISBN 0-86656-821-2. ISBN 0-86656-854-9 (pbk.)
    1. Aged—Health and hygiene. 2. Exercise for the aged. I. Title.
RA777.6.W45   1988
613'.0438—dc19

88-23326
CIP

ISBN 13: 978-1-315-86413-6 (ebk)
ISBN 13: 978-0-86656-854-8 (pbk)

Dedication

This book is dedicated to mankind:
To the weak, the strong, the infirmed, and the healthy.
For all mankind to remember,
To respect life.

To care for yourself and others.

To be loving in all your ways.

      and

To change your life and the world begins with you today!

This book is also dedicated to the memory of my father, Emil Weiss, who died on August 8, 1986, 6 days before his 65th birthday.

The "Feeling Great!" Wellness Program for Older Adults

CONTENTS

Preface

Within the following pages I try to recreate the magic of the "Feeling Great!" program—the liveliness in the air, the spark in the participants' eyes, the sound of their laughter and talking. This book is designed to give the reader a glimpse of an exciting and vital program.

It is a program of everyday miracles—the regaining of body movement and the expanding of each persons' physical abilities. A program that helps in developing peer relationships and offers supportive guidance which creates a feeling of emotional wellness. A program where senior citizens experience a sense of wellness in their mind, body and spirit beyond their perceived and daily "ritual-bound" limits. Through the program, participants gain a new arena of social supports which culminate in new friendships, better relationships, an increased sense of self-esteem, and a feeling of purpose to get up everyday and make it "Feel Great."

This book is created for people who desire and are willing to strive for a "richer" life. Older adults have the ability to reach their full potential in health, fitness, and well-being at any age. This includes feeling good about themselves—vital, vibrant, and having the ability to overcome barriers of ill health, poor diet, sedentary lifestyle, and physical and emotional difficulties.

The "Feeling Great!" program helps older adults to learn about staying in shape; physically, emotionally, and spiritually. This process is solidified by the individual's commitment, reinforced in the program, and guided by personal action to respect, care for, and honor their own and others' well-being.

The participants are empowered to become teachers of their generation through sharing their knowledge with their peers, relatives, and the community in general. They become teachers in learning how to live a life in peace, harmony, joy, and good health.

A life to celebrate
A life to share with others
A life in recognition and fulfillment of oneself.

Senior citizens must now take the time to impart the wisdom of their years, the strength gained through their experiences, and the refinement of their inner senses. It is also a time for seniors to learn how to live gracefully and vigorously keeping their body, mind, and spirit in top form. As individuals growing older, they call to action their strength, willpower, and love. This task of life is to be all we can be, to the best of our ability. Older adults must not succumb to negativity, depression, and illness but rise to affirm that life is good, they make a difference, and they can live healthy strong active lives all of their days.

Acknowledgements

The "Feeling Great!" program has been developed with the help and guidance of the Lee Circle YMCA staff in New Orleans, LA. A note of appreciation goes out to Howard Leighton, Jo Ann Moinet, and Betsy Teuton for their support and assistance in the development of the program.

Thanks to Julianna Padgett, Isabel Messina, Jewell Knobloch, and to my wife Faith Weiss for their great editing assistance. Thanks are also extended to Richard Vallon, Jr. for his fine photographic contribution, to C. Jessie Jones, PhD, for her contributing material, to Hugh S. Mellert, MPA, for his aid in health care resources, and to Steve Winn for his assistance on the computer.

Special thanks go to all of the participants of the "Feeling Great!" program who made this book come alive through their commitment to their well-being, as exemplified in the "Feeling Great!" program.

Chapter I

Introduction
to the
"Feeling Great!" Program

BIRTH OF THE "FEELING GREAT!" PROGRAM:
ONE INSTRUCTOR'S CHALLENGE

I never liked to exercise, I never liked to sweat, I never liked to run, I never joined an exercise class, except in my youth when I played tennis throughout the summers. Professionally, I have worked for over ten years as an art therapist and counselor specializing in working with older adults. When I worked long hours, sometimes two jobs plus private clients, I tried to make sure I ate well for nourishment but I often became worn down and tired. I was accustomed to overworking and not taking care of myself, while taking care of others.

In New Orleans, Louisiana as an art therapist and counselor I spent a few years working on a consultation/short-term contract basis with two other people in a program called Longevity Therapy. Longevity Therapy is a motivational program designed for staff and older adults of senior citizen centers, senior apartment complexes, and nursing homes. Group activities for seniors focused on using the arts such as movement, expressive art, and music to elicit feelings and thoughts and generate dialogue, insight, and group sharing. The program sensitizes staff members to the psycho-social-physical needs of senior citizens and their options. Our goal was to bring about a positive long-term change in the milieu.

Bobbie Graubarth-Syzller, founder of Longevity Therapy is a woman in her 60s who believes that movement is an essential aspect of maintaining a healthy sense of self. She led the Longevity Therapy movement experiences which were most energetic and inspiring. Bobbie was able to pick up the spirits of everyone in the group and bring out the best in people. The senior citizens responded in an overwhelming manner to the movement experiences, loving to touch, play, move around, and obtain a greater sense of feeling for their bodies. I found that the movement experiences could motivate people who were stiff and silent to "wake them up" and "bring them to their senses." This process enabled them to reach out and express themselves. I assisted Bobbie in many movement activities and it made me more aware and interested in the power of movement and exercise for aiding the well-being of individuals.

In our group discussions, it struck me how alienated these older adults often felt about their body. They talked about losing weight but few went on diets and stayed on them to produce the results they sought. In the group discussions many people would joke about going on diets or exercising. Though it seemed that they would have loved to lose weight and get into better shape by exercising, these goals did not feel like a reality to these people. They did not have the resources, group support or guidance in these areas. I began to realize that they felt their body was not under their full control. They felt unable to keep their body in shape and at the mercy of medications for their arthritis and other physical complaints. They did not have the "tools" or teachers to learn about exercise, proper diet and nutrition, and the special health needs of older adults, nor did they have a supportive environment to nurture their health needs.

I saw a major problem here. The primary and possibly only person these people had to discuss their health concerns and needs with was their doctor who at times could not give them the time and instruction they needed. I also realized our workshops over a six-month period—twice a week were not going to fully address the participants needs in exercise and health education. Rather, I felt they needed a program they could attend on a regular basis, two or three times a week.

I remembered in my years of counseling older adults in mental health clinics in New York, California, and West Virginia how many people felt distressed about their physical condition. Often, they were depressed and seemed to feel they had few options besides going to their doctor and getting different medications. For these individuals, their problems seemed to be a revolving door with no exit. I thought that their depression may have to do with a sense of lack of control in their lives. And I speculated to myself, if we offered a good health education, exercise, and peer support program, how many people who were depressed or had other emotional problems would find some relief, learn better coping skills, and begin to get better. My speculation evolved into the "Feeling Great!" program, a pilot project of Lee Circle YMCA.

Around the time I was formulating these ideas I met Howard Leighton, program director of the local YMCA. Through our conversation he mentioned that the YMCA did not have an exercise program for senior citizens and they would like to offer one to the community. I was appalled that the YMCA had programs for every other population but lacked programs for senior citizens. I told him that I thought it was vital to the community to have a good exercise and health education program for senior citizens and described the ease with which such a program could be designed. He was very interested. I stipulated that the YMCA would need to train me to be an exercise instructor before I would conduct the program.

With my ideas concerning the needs of older adults for health education, peer support, and exercise in order to regain their lost health or continue living with vitality, I designed the "Feeling Great!" program. The YMCA liked my design and offered me a part-time position (twenty hours a week) to conduct the program. The YMCA agreed to privately train me in fitness through their staff. They also sent me to various workshops to be certified as an exercise instructor and in other YMCA program certifications.

I was stuck. I thought to myself in amazement, how was I, a person who always hated exercise, going to be trained as an exercise instructor to lead programs and motivate older adults in health promotion? Then I thought, I might be the best instructor because of my dislike for exercise. Like many senior citizens, I needed to improve my physical condition, and learning and teaching about exercise seemed to be the best way to begin. I believe the teacher should always be the best student. I decided that if in my stubbornness, I could enjoy exercising and improve my health, then any older person who had an aversion to exercise could also like it and gain from the program. This opportunity presented a great challenge to me. One of my goals was to set up one of the finest programs in the country where senior citizens would be able to obtain health care information and resources, have a place to exercise, meet their friends, and do new and exciting things together as a supportive peer group.

With my sense of entrepreneurship, I enjoyed designing and setting up the program. I made contacts with local hospitals and health care professionals for health care information and wrote to national organizations such as AARP for pamphlets on various health topics. The marketing department of the YMCA assisted me in designing the brochure and informational materials I needed. I gave presentations on exercise and the "Feeling Great!" program throughout the city at senior citizen centers, senior apartment complexes, and other senior citizen groups and organizations. I listed the program under community events in the newspapers and had community service spots aired on the television and radio. Also, at the same time to get into better shape, I began an exercise program of jogging every other day.

The marketing department of the YMCA contacted a radio station about the program, who responded by asking me to be on a morning talk show. The show was at 6:00 a.m. and I was sure no one was up at that time. But to my amazement, I got more responses from the radio show than from my other endeavors. I found out that many senior citizens wake up early and listen to the radio! Whenever I presented talks about the program in the community, the audience usually responded in a very favorable manner, but only a few participants would be interested enough to come to the class. Using the media, radio, television, and newspapers, I reached a much larger audience and even though my presentation was much shorter, sometimes only a matter of minutes, my efforts seemed to be more fruitful than my personal lectures. I really enjoyed public speaking and gave many lectures to groups all around New Orleans, but for advertising the program most efficiently, I had to focus on mass media publicity.

My first "Feeling Great!" class had only five people but over time the program really grew. By word of mouth the notice of the class spread around town. A breakthrough for the program came when WWL-TV (Channel Four) did a five minute news spot on the "Feeling Great!" program which brought many new participants. Six months later WDSU-TV (Channel Six) did a news/human interest spot on the program and we became even more popular. The teachers in public schools began hearing about the program and in the summers, many older teachers would attend the class. In the meantime whenever we had a special event such as the first and second year anniversary of the program, we received significant coverage in the local newspapers along with pictures of participants and testimonials about the program.

An interesting experience happened to me through my participation in the program. I began to really enjoy exercising. I found that I had more energy, felt better about myself, and found myself to be a more effective counselor and art therapist. I was clearer in my thinking and stronger in my work than ever before. Strangely, for some reason I even found my hearing improved. The program ended up to be the biggest gift I could give to myself, my own good health.

In the second year of conducting the program my father, Emil Weiss, died of a heart attack at age 64. I realized that since I worked like my father, continuously 6 to 7 days a week, I was headed for the same fate if I did not continue exercising and eating in a healthy manner.

After the first year of conducting the program I held a staff training workshop for the staff of other local YMCAs. Most YMCA staff were very interested in conducting a program similar to the "Feeling Great!" program. Some people said that they could not get enough time in the gym or they did not have enough time to develop such a comprehensive program. But others started a program based on the "Feeling Great!" model. I offered them the use of the "Feeling Great!" program name, but interestingly enough, people made up their own names for their programs. Later I realized that it was probably best that they created their own names for their programs. I believe the program is the instructor, he/she is totally responsible for the program and should develop a name that suits his/her personality, YMCA, and population.

I have heard good things about the programs which were set up by the staff I trained. But also, another very important goal I had was to teach senior citizens to conduct exercise/health education programs themselves. With my encouragement, many participants of the "Feeling Great!" program have begun teaching exercises and sharing their health care literature and knowledge with their family and friends. I hope that one day we will have senior citizens conducting daily quality exercise/health education programs in every long-term care setting, community center/senior citizens center, senior citizen apartment complex, and wherever senior citizens congregate. It is my hope that through this program older adults will be motivated to learn and share with their peers the knowledge of how to master their lives, overcoming the obstacles they face, and continuing to grow healthy and strong everyday.

PROGRAM DESCRIPTION

The "Feeling Great!" program is for people over the age of fifty who want to maintain a feeling of physical and emotional well-being or who want to recover a healthy feeling of body and mind through a structured wellness program. The program provides participants with learning and practice in proper exercise, relaxation techniques, health care lectures/discussions, enjoyable group activities, and an optional swimming and/or water exercise period. "Feeling Great!" classes are held two or three times a week on an ongoing basis. Participants can join the program at any time, and either pay for one session, a week, or a month depending on their preference.

"Feeling Great!" guides participants in learning about healthy ways of living through health education and exercise, and offers a supportive enriching milieu to learn and share with one's peers. It encourages peer support and provides motivational talks on the value and importance of having a positive attitude along with group discussions on health, fitness, and the psycho-social-physical changes encountered in aging. It aids participants in making realistic commitments to their personal health care program and helps them in meeting their desired goals.

Most importantly, the "Feeling Great!" program provides a

good healthy workout for participants, enabling each person to progress at his or her own pace. Exercises are taught which can be done at home with common objects such as broomsticks, small weights, rubber tubing or towels, and frisbees. Home exercise programs are outlined by the instructor to fit each participant's needs. For optimal benefit, home exercises should be done on a regular basis, everyday or every other day along with consistent participation in the program.

"FEELING GREAT!" APPROACH

The "Feeling Great!" program teaches that a person is either part of the problem or part of the solution. No one stands still. We are either aware of and responsive to our bodies' physical/nutritional/ and emotional needs or else we are acting irresponsibly by not acknowledging our basic needs for healthy living.

For example, the "Feeling Great!" program instructs participants about good eating habits and the nutritional value of foods as well as those foods to limit in one's diet. Proper exercise is stressed to help participants stay in good physical shape to meet the changing physical conditions of middle age and of older adulthood. Exercises such as range of motion, flexibility, strengthening, and endurance are used for total fitness. The program reinforces the importance of having a healthy attitude with which to approach the experiences and stresses of daily life.

The "Feeling Great!" concept of wellness does not mean only eating correctly and exercising, but rather a balanced healthy lifestyle reflecting a respect, awareness, and responsibility to the needs of the mind, body, and spirit. While teaching the importance of emotional and physical wellness, participants are reminded that new health problems may sometimes be created by compulsively exercising and dieting. Moderation and balance in diet, exercise, and lifestyle is vital for a healthy sense of well-being.

An important reminder to participants is that occasional exercise will only provide occasional benefit. Exercising regularly will provide consistent and progressive benefits to the body. Similar to a diet, if you do not stick to it, you will not achieve the desired results. An occasional healthy meal will only supply you with the proper nutrition occasionally. Regular exercise, healthy diet, and a positive to approach to life provide the ingredients for "Feeling Great!" everyday.

Though the "Feeling Great!" program was initiated in a YMCA, it can be taught in numerous settings. However, it is recommended that the program instructor take advantage of the high quality leadership training provided by YMCAs throughout the country (see page 132 for more information on Fitness Leadership).

Program Methods

1. Practice correct ways of exercising:
    - cardiovascular fitness
    - stretching with full range of motion
    - muscle strength and endurance exercises
    - balance and agility exercises
    - coordination exercises
    - breathing exercises
    - relaxation techniques
2. By means of group discussions/lectures teach about health education and a healthy attitude toward life, including ways to deal effectively with the circumstances of one's life.
3. Encourage peer support and relationships through class interaction.

Program Goals

1. To increase fitness, health, and general well-being.
2. To increase physical, social, and psychological awareness of self.
3. To teach participants how to provide better self-care—physically, socially, and psychologically.
4. To teach participants how to reduce minor tensions and body aches through exercise and relaxation, and how to stay in good physical shape.

5. To provide a structured exercise program which participants can do at home to supplement their "Feeling Great!" classes.
6. To provide a community based program which offers peer support along with health education, a vital exercise program, and a recreational outlet.
7. To help participants develop new abilities and to regain those which are dormant due to lack of exercise.
8. To address the needs of the whole person — mind, body and spirit; the social, psychological, spiritual, and physical aspects of the person.

   a. *Social* — To develop new relationships, share in meaningful dialogue, gain intimacy with others, and have friends to go to social events with.
   b. *Psychological* — To learn to cope with the difficulties of life, develop new interests and hobbies, "retire" to a new and more interesting "occupation" — the occupation of fulfilling oneself.
   c. *Spiritual* — To gain strength from one's faith, perform service for one's fellow man and one's community, etc.
   d. *Physical* — To take the best care possible of one's body through exercise, diet/nutrition, proper use of medications, and preventive health care.

ADDRESSING THE NEEDS OF THE "WHOLE" PERSON

In addressing the needs of the whole person, the mind, body and spirit have to be taken into account, and responsibly loved, nurtured, and developed. This includes the social, psychological, physical, and spiritual aspects of the self. Instructors cannot assume that participants are already aware of the depth and beauty of the dimensions of the self and the needs experienced in the maturation process of aging. Rather, instructors and participants must fully examine and explore this spectrum of qualities in the development of the individual. Furthermore, we must discover what it means to experience the maturation of self-actualization and fulfillment of the individual. A true wellness program needs to sufficiently address itself to the above noted areas to succinctly and comprehensively aid people in a balanced self-growth program.

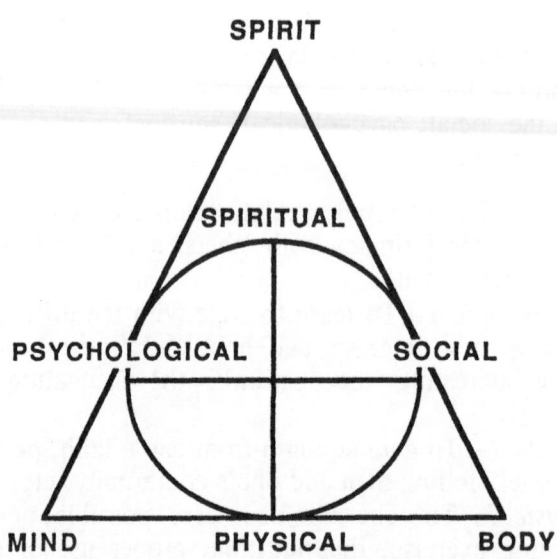

MARKETING SUGGESTIONS

In marketing the program always keep in mind the program's objective: to provide an ongoing wellness program for adults and senior citizens which includes health education, various types of exercises (sitting, standing, and mat exercises), water exercises and swimming, motivation and peer support, recreational group activities, and teaching relaxation techniques.

Target Groups

The program is offered to men and women fifty years of age and older (age requirement is flexible, upon request people in their 40s are allowed to join). Classes can be formed with people from:

- Senior Citizen apartment complexes
- Senior Citizen Centers
- Nursing homes
- Senior social clubs, e.g., AARP, New Orleans Recreation Department — "Golden Agers," religious groups
- Community members

Before beginning the program all participants must obtain either verbal or written permission from their doctor. It is recommended that participants ask their doctors for a letter stating any exercise they should avoid due to their physical condition, medications, physical disabilities, and/or previous accidents or surgeries. Also, participants must sign the informed consent registration form which is located on the program brochure, page 191. The informed consent notes the individual's responsibility for their physical well-being while participating in the "Feeling Great!" program.

Marketing Keys

1. Advertise through newspaper articles describing the program, participants, special events of the program such as anniversary parties and participants' accomplishments.
2. Radio talk shows to interview participants and the exercise instructor about the program.
3. Public service announcements on television, radio, and listing in newspapers under community events and the sports section.
4. Have a health fair geared to older adults utilizing the community hospitals support for staff to volunteer their services.
5. Create tee-shirts with the program logo for all participants, family members, and friends of the program — it's great for publicity and group morale. Your participants are your best advertisers — word of mouth by a trusted source is a golden key to older adults.
6. The exercise instructor can promote the program through giving talks on the importance of exercise and handing out flyers and brochures about the program at nursing homes, senior citizen centers, adult day care centers, senior citizen apartment complexes, AARP groups, religious organizations, and other community wide senior citizen groups. Some facilities may provide transportation to the program for its members.

7. Hand out flyers/brochures at the local YMCA and other health clubs for members' relatives, friends, or acquaintances. People who are already interested in health and fitness recognize its value and importance to the older adult and they can recommend the program to others.
8. For promotion, advertise that a free "Feeling Great!" class and exercise booklet are given to new participants. In encouraging good attendance it is helpful to offer class specials such as when participants bring a friend both people receive a free class, or participants who come for four consecutive weeks receive a free class.

INGREDIENTS WHICH MAKE THE "FEELING GREAT!" PROGRAM SPECIAL

1. The program provides a complete workout, a meaningful social outlet, a health education lecture/discussion and a fun recreational activity within one session. Sufficient time is allocated for each activity within the session to provide participants with a sense of satisfaction and accomplishment.
2. A mutual feeling among participants of caring, support, and togetherness.
3. A feeling of love, acceptance, and fun in the group.
4. Regardless of physical disability or emotional difficulty each person is accepted by the class with feelings of hope, enthusiasm, and encouragement.
5. Participants of varying physical abilities are able to exercise together, receive a good work-out, and contribute to the program by either physically or verbally helping others in their exercises or showing new exercise routines they have discovered.
6. Bi-weekly social activities are held after the exercise session which enable participants to get to know each other better, build friendships, and have fun with their peers. A few of the social activities participants enjoy are: dining out, visiting a museum, seeing a movie.
7. The recognition of the spiritual aspects of life and the strength received from faith. As a reflection of our commitment to our spiritual beliefs, we discuss the ways in which we make a contri-

bution to others through volunteering our time and helping out where needed.

8. Group discussions and health lectures in each session on psycho-social-physical issues and problems facing older adults. These discussions give participants a chance to share their concerns and learn new ways of dealing with life.

9. The program has caring, trained, and certified instructors who are knowledgeable of the psycho-social-physical issues facing older adults and who are supportive of participants in helping them to develop their abilities to their potential.

WHY PEOPLE NEED THE "FEELING GREAT!" PROGRAM

1. Many older people do not feel comfortable in a regular aerobic or exercise program. They may be ashamed of their bodies and of being out of shape, especially when they are with people who are in much better physical condition. Also, most aerobic and exercise programs are usually geared to younger people who are in better physical condition and the programs are often conducted at a fast and rigorous pace. This type of exercise class climate can intimidate older people preventing them from taking enough time to work up to the class level.

   The "Feeling Great!" program begins at a slow to moderate pace and helps participants to gradually develop their physical fitness. Most older people feel more comfortable if they are exercising with their peers and able to progress at a comfortable rate.

2. Due to the increasingly sedentary lifestyles of many senior citizens, most older people need to learn a daily exercise program to do at home. This program can help them keep their bodies flexible and in good shape, aiding in reducing the pain of arthritis and other physical ailments they may incur.

3. The program helps participants improve their stability, agility, and mobility, thereby reducing possible falls and accidents.

4. The program teaches stress reduction and relaxation techniques to help people who have trouble sleeping (reduce the use of sleeping medications) and to aid those in physical pain. It also

teaches ways to deal with the stresses of daily life which seem to increase with age as people encounter more losses in their life.

5. Health education and preventive medicine are taught which are essential ingredients in "learning how to stay well."
6. The program provides an enjoyable social activity for older adults with their peers. Also, participants develop leadership skills through assisting in leading exercises, group discussions, and planning and organizing field trips.
7. The program aids and motivates people in independent living through improving their physical condition, increasing social contacts, developing new relationships, and learning more about various community-wide opportunities and events through field trips and group discussions.
8. The program helps to increase the quality of people's lives through good preventive health care and thereby reduce or slow down the possible psychological, social, and physical deteriorating aspects of the aging process.

BENEFITS OF THE PROGRAM ACTIVITIES

1. *Sitting, standing, and movement exercises* develop good posture, improve joint mobility, and promote the correct way to walk, sit, stand, and to get down onto a mat.
2. *Balancing and coordination exercises* help to prevent falls and to become steadier on their feet.
3. *Breathing and cardiovascular exercises* increase endurance and enable participants to have more energy to do things.
4. *Range of motion and flexibility exercises* help to aid in preventing further arthritic deterioration in regard to limitations of joint rotation and help to increase flexibility and movement.
5. *Endurance and strengthening exercises* help in toning up and strengthening key postural muscles.
6. *Reflex exercises and coordination activities* aid in coordination and agility, providing more effective and easier use of body movement.
7. *Water exercises* help to aid in preventing further arthritic deterioration in regard to limitations of joint rotation and help to increase flexibility and movement. They also relieve stress on

weight bearing joints which then offers a greater freedom of movement.

8. *Swimming* provides the same benefits described in number seven, plus aids in toning up the body and in endurance through the cardiovascular activity of swimming. Psychologically, learning to swim helps participants increase confidence in their abilities.
9. *General exercise* helps in digestion, sleeping, and body movement.
10. *Relaxation exercises* aid in sleeping problems, in reducing and coping with stress, and help to lower blood pressure.
11. *Health lectures* aid in learning how best to take care of the body, physically and emotionally, through information on diet, nutrition, medical check-ups, healthy patterns of living, preventive medicine, and a variety of other related topics.
12. *Group activities and the total program* aid in physical fitness; assist in independent living; help in overcoming depression, isolation, loneliness; aid in reducing stress; improve peer relationships and provide peer support; increase self-esteem; and promote having fun with others.

WHAT A SUCCESSFUL PROGRAM WILL MEAN!

1. It will change people's lives enabling them to become healthier, more fit, able to take better care of themselves.
2. It provides a healthy, social, community-based outlet so needed by many middle-aged and older adults.
3. It is an educational resource/learning center providing information on nutrition, fitness, health tips, and a range of other topics pertinent to the older adult.
4. It will aid people in endurance, strength, and flexibility enabling them to be more active in their lives and experience a wider spectrum of opportunities and life enjoyments.
5. It will provide a structured program for people to learn exercises to do at home to guard against the problems encountered by the effects of a sedentary lifestyle.
6. It will aid individuals who have physical problems in regaining their strength, flexibility, and endurance through appropriate

exercise and it will motivate them to stay active and independent.

7. It will help people improve their sense of balance and agility, thus helping prevent falls, and it will promote their confidence in their physical abilities.
8. It can help people who have sleep or digestion problems through exercising and learning relaxation techniques.
9. It can aid people's mental faculties through stimulating discussions, learning, and peer interaction.
10. It can be one of the most important programs participants will have a chance to join. Enabling senior citizens to learn how to take good care of themselves will help them attain good physical, emotional, and psychological health and will enhance their life.
11. The program is a step toward beginning a "University for the Second Phase of Life," a place for adults to learn how to live well at any age.

We are either part of the problem or part of the solution.

Let's be part of the solution.

Chapter II

The "Feeling Great!" Class Members

The "Feeling Great!" group is a class where people walk in feeling 70 years old, possibly tired and weary, and can walk out feeling vibrant and youthful. It is a class in which people learn to give up their canes and wheelchairs, to feel confident and able to walk correctly on their own. A multifaceted group full of fun and pleasure, lots of joking, sometimes hard exercising, and sometimes taking it easy — a place to forget your troubles or share your concerns with others, a place to make new friends, to have a good time and just to be yourself.

One of the many rewarding aspects of the "Feeling Great!" program is the camaraderie and respect found between participants. This includes the enjoyment of meeting new friends, discussing social and health-related issues, going out together, being a support for each other, exercising and letting go of the stresses of the day. For members, the group becomes a place to share intimate feelings, thoughts, and concerns with others who have similar experiences.

Unfortunately, a large number of older people today have lost many social supports and feel isolated with a lack of resources. This includes a loss of meaningful social contact. The "Feeling Great!" program addresses these needs and concerns of the older adult.

What makes the "Feeling Great!" program so wonderful is the initiative many older people take in the program. They volunteer to set up the exercise room, call participants who are sick and to remind others to diet, exercise, and attend class and field trips. Some volunteers become resource people to help find and organize interesting field trips. Other volunteers sometimes conduct the health-lecture or exercise portion of the class. With the help of the participants, the group becomes a vital support to the mental health and well-being of everyone involved.

Volunteering enables participants to take on a new responsibility that brings with it a sense of pride and self-worth. New possibilities are created for these individuals by discovering their strengths, abilities, and new enjoyments. People who feel lost in a system of retirement, disability, and "survival living" on a limited income have a chance to make a difference among their peers in a vital health care program.

Each member of the class is a delegate for the program, recruiting new members and sharing valuable health care pamphlets and information with family and friends. Like a pebble dropped in a lake, the ripples affect many people far and wide.

To give the reader a more intimate feeling of the group, participants were interviewed, sharing their personal experience of the class. The class has been filmed for television news, reported often in the local newspapers, but the full story is held in the experience of the participants' lives.

AUGUST WILLIAMS

Mrs. Williams called to ask if her husband who was 67 years old and recovering from a car accident could participate in the "Feeling Great!" program. Due to the accident he had undergone an operation for a damaged vertebrae in his neck. His right side was partially paralyzed and he walked with a limp, assisted by the use of a cane.

She explained that since the accident he had been very depressed. He was always a hard worker and a very busy man. The thought of not being able to work and be active upset him considerably. He did not know what to do with all of his free time or with his life. He felt very uncomfortable at Senior Citizen Centers because he could not relate to congregating with seniors just to eat, talk, and do handicrafts. I told Mrs. Williams that I thought he would enjoy our program because the exercises would help his physical condition, the health lecture discussions were very stimulating and interesting, and we have a lively, fun group. I explained that with his doctor's consent he could come to the "Feeling Great!" program and I would monitor his activity and assist him in learning the proper exercise for his condition.

August (Mr. Williams) began coming regularly to the program

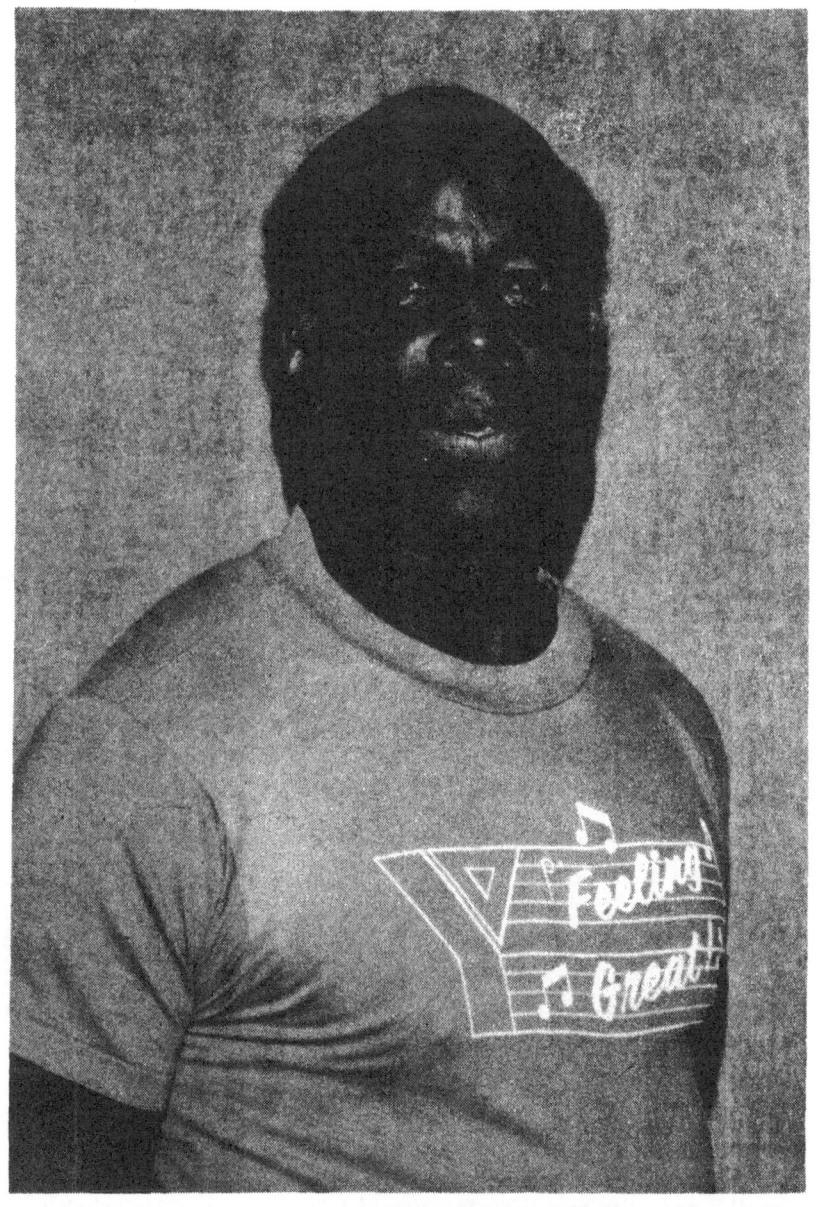

August Williams

and really enjoyed it, especially the camaraderie and support he received from fellow members. Other participants took an interest in helping August to learn the exercise routines and would motivate and encourage him to stay with the program and exercises. In class he often got frustrated because he was not able to do many of the exercises due to his limited physical abilities at the time. He had trouble walking, standing up straight, straightening out and moving his right arm and leg.

After a month of participating in the class I realized that August needed a more concentrated physical activity program to help him rehabilitate. We discussed the benefits of becoming a member of the YMCA so he could workout three times a week on the exercise machines, go walking on the jogging track, and still come to the "Feeling Great!" program (the program is free to members of the YMCA). August was inspired by the other class members who joined the YMCA to use the center's full facilities. So he decided it would be in his best interests to join. He began to come to the "Y" three times a week, for two and a half hours each day. When it was convenient he also attended the "Feeling Great!" class and participated in the socials and special events.

The program director at the YMCA designed an exercise program for August using various exercise machines to help bring back the full function in his muscles and to increase his coordination, range of motion, and overall physical abilities. August was very faithful to his exercise routine. After a year and a half of exercising he no longer needed to rely on using his cane. He regained full function of his body except for a slight limited movement in his right wrist. He is now able to walk with good posture and even run. Previous to his accident he was always a nervous person with high blood pressure, but ever since he began exercising regularly he doesn't feel nervous anymore. His doctor told him that he no longer has high blood pressure. August was sold on exercising and treasured the companionship of his fellow members at the YMCA.

Due to August's great achievement in his physical fitness he was able to go back to work, giving him a sense of pride and self-esteem. August was a role model for participants in the "Feeling Great!" program and they felt proud to be a part of his rehabilitation. A man who once told the group "No, I just can't do those exercises" is a person who achieved more than he ever dreamed possible. August is a living testament to the potential we each possess which can be unlocked through our efforts and motivation along with support from others.

DORIS OLMSTED

Doris was living alone in an apartment in Los Angeles, recently retired at age 83 from selling real estate to Hollywood customers, when her son called her to suggest that she should move to New Orleans. He felt that she would be safer and happier living closer to him.

Doris had previously fallen twice in her own home and broken both hips, in which steel pins were inserted. In 1984 she cracked the left side of her rib cage in another fall. Due to her recent physical difficulties and wanting to see her son, she agreed to move to New Orleans. On July 15, 1985 Doris's son called to tell her to start packing because he had found her an apartment in New Orleans which she needed to move into by August 1, 1985.

Doris came to New Orleans feeling displaced and depressed. She missed the cool weather by the beaches of California and was shocked by the hot, humid weather of New Orleans. Away from her friends, familiar surroundings, and the social life she knew and developed from over thirty years in Los Angeles she was a stranger in a strange land, New Orleans, with no friends, no acquaintances, just her son, Clint. Her son was a member of the Lee Circle YMCA, and at one time a participant in the "Feeling Great!" program. As soon as Doris came to New Orleans he encouraged her to participate in the "Feeling Great!" program.

Doris at age 84, suffering from severe arthritis, feeling depressed, having trouble walking, put on a smile and came to the "Feeling Great!" program. She started off slowly, but gradually improved in her walking, became more steady on her feet, and learned to walk briskly. Her range of motion in her arms and hands increased, and from the finger exercises she was now able once again to play piano, a pleasure she had not been able to do for many

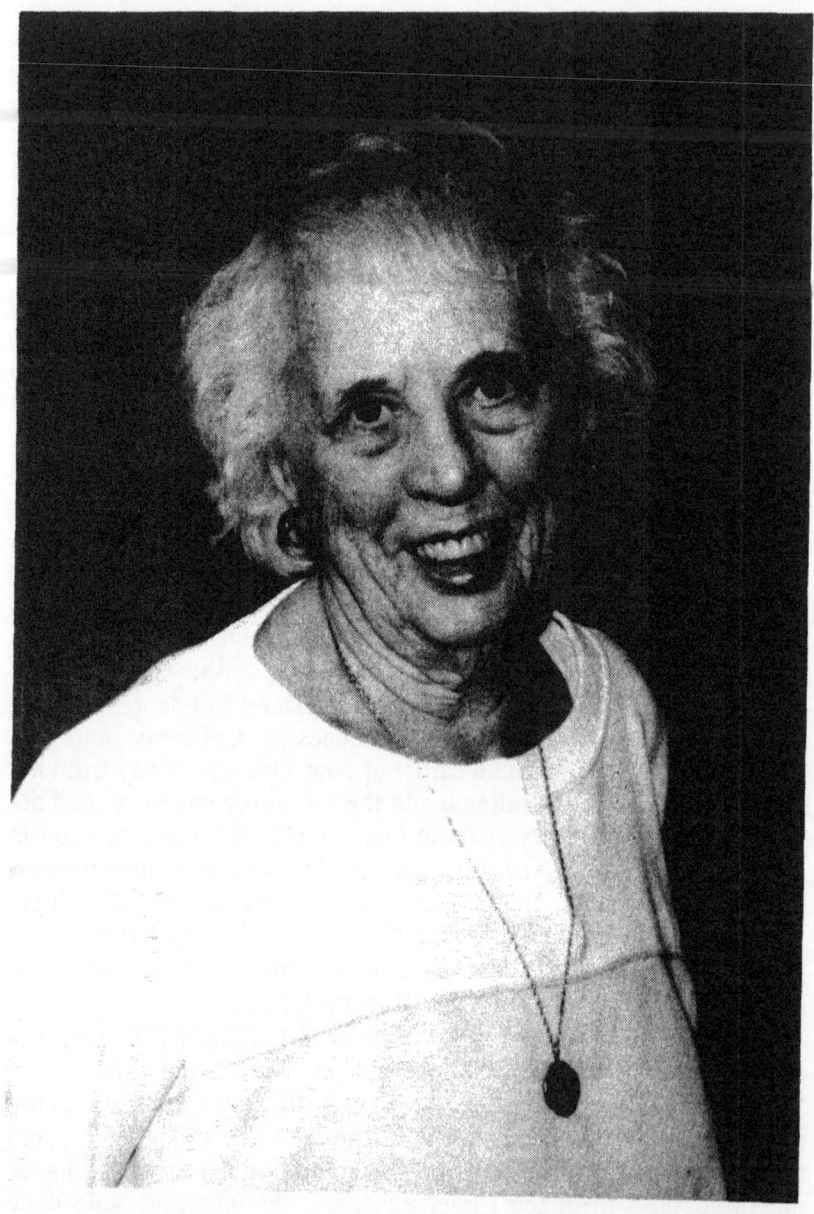

Doris Olmsted

years. She became more flexible and relaxed throughout her whole body, reducing arthritic pain in her joints. She also enjoyed the social activities that the program offered her. She made many new friends in the class and began going to restaurants, attending social teas, and participating in field trips with members of the "Feeling Great!" class. After the first couple of months in the program she exclaimed that she felt her mind cleared up, and no longer felt depressed.

From the experience of participating in the "Feeling Great!" program Doris was able to make a successful, enjoyable adjustment to her new home in New Orleans, finding new friends, a social outlet, and getting to know the city she now calls home. She claims that due to the exercise program she now feels physically better than she had in decades.

Doris's personal philosophy is to have a positive outlook on life and to take each day as it comes. This attitude and her way of life has made her a great inspiration and "teacher" to the class. She has meant so much to the class members that they gave her a special party for her 85th birthday. Her life has been an example for others, showing how we can achieve our goal of "Feeling Great!" every day with some enjoyable exercise, friendly socializing and a positive attitude toward life.

GLORY KIEFFER

At age 67 Glory retired after 15 years of working for the Council On Aging as a Homemaker, helping senior citizens. She always enjoyed helping others, meeting new people and socializing, but when she retired she was looking for new outlets and interesting activities to participate in. Her apartment building is only a few blocks from the YMCA and in the first month of the program I gave a talk about the "Feeling Great!" program at the monthly apartment building meeting. Upon hearing my lecture, she immediately joined the program. She was always interested in exercising and wanted to meet new people.

After a couple of months in the program Glory volunteered to help make the class refreshments, set out the exercise equipment

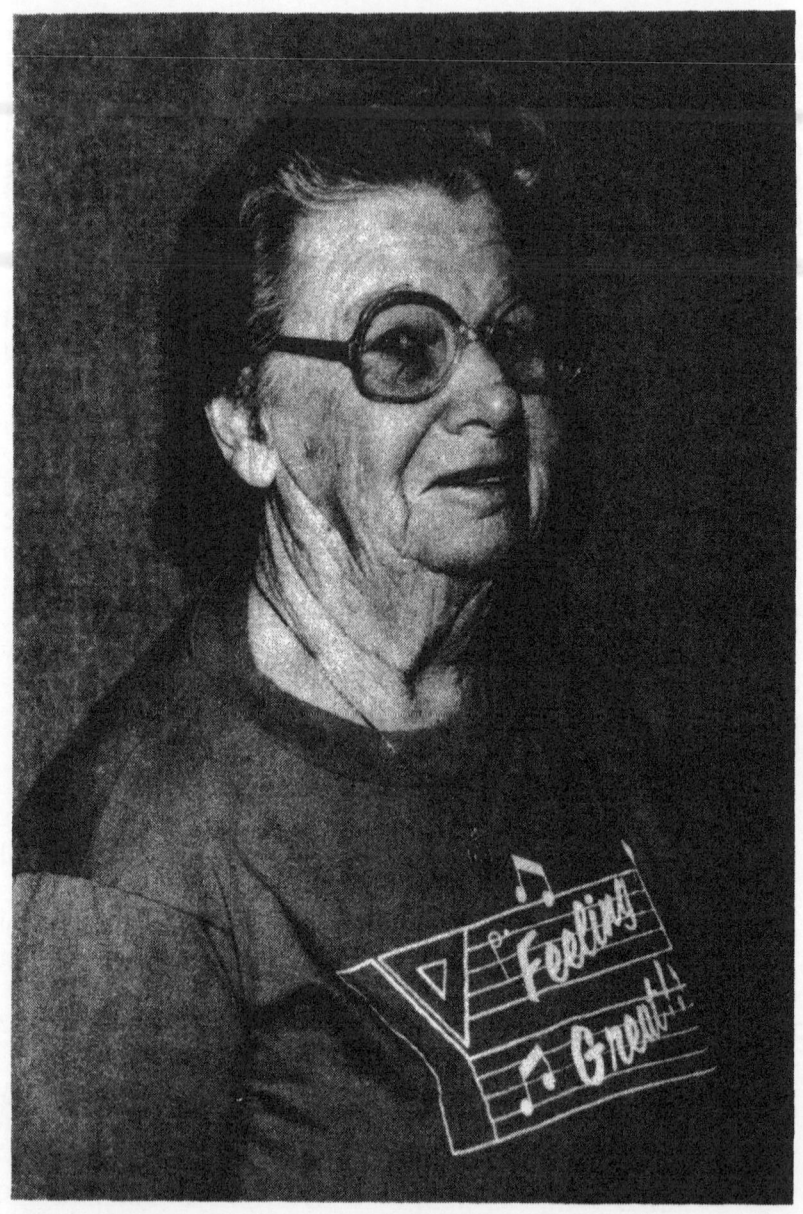

Glory Kieffer

and to help out in any way needed. Her assistance allowed me to spend more time with the new participants and to talk with the regulars in the program. Being a volunteer gave her a tremendous feeling of being needed and doing something constructive, gaining respect and appreciation from her peers. She became friends with everyone in the program and a whole new social life opened up to her. In the health lecture discussions she had an opportunity to share her feelings and concerns about her retirement and the daily difficulties of life, along with the successful life changes and adjustments she has made.

As time went on Glory began to express more of herself, and became more relaxed, spontaneous, and flexible in the group. She would poke fun at the instructor, tell jokes, and get everyone in an old-time sing-along with songs like "Pennies From Heaven" at the end of the group. She became the sunlight in the group making everyone's day a little brighter. She really knew how to make the group come alive and everyone loved her for it.

The other side of Glory was that at one time in her life she had some personal difficulties which she overcame with the help of the organization Recovery, Inc. She now volunteers for Recovery, Inc. and conducts weekly groups for people in emotional crisis. The wisdom she gained from dealing with her personal difficulties she freely shares with others who are distressed. Informal peer counseling and peer support is one of the essential aspects of the "Feeling Great!" program which Glory adds to immensely.

Glory attended the program regularly for over two years, rarely missing a class. Every week she looks forward to coming to the group for her own health and well-being and to give her an opportunity to help others, fulfilling the "social worker-compassionate" aspect of herself. Glory says that the "Feeling Great!" program helps her physically and mentally and gives her as much as she gets from the program. She claims the class has made her feel younger and just "Feel Great!"

FRANCES STAKELUM

Frances, age 77, is a widow who retired in 1977 after working for 37 years in the paint and varnish business. Between 1977 and 1985

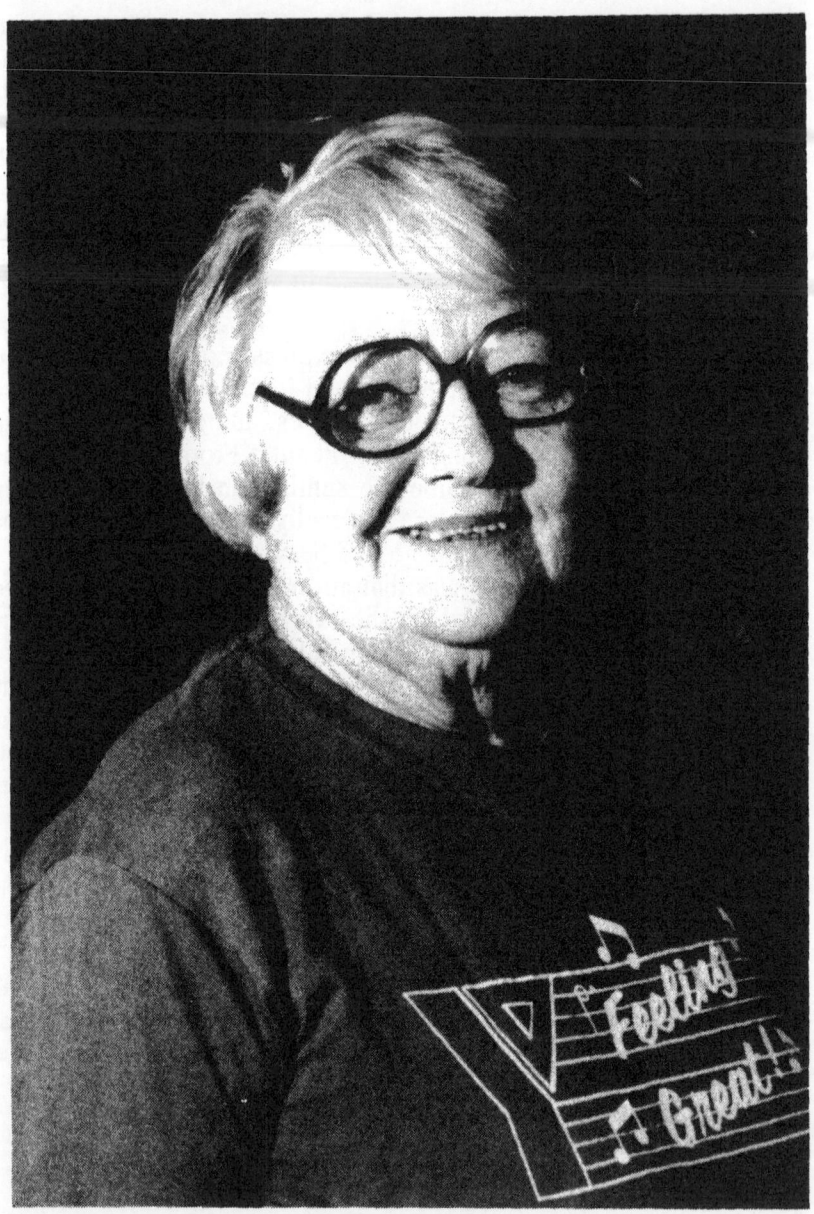

Frances Stakelum

she stayed home, slept often, and rarely went anywhere. She became so stiff from inactivity that she was not even able to raise her leg to get into a bus. When New Orleans hosted the 1984 World's Fair she was not able to attend because she couldn't walk two blocks before becoming exhausted. Also, on Mardi Gras day she was not able to walk a few blocks to see the parades. Frances was depressed, living alone, and feeling that she couldn't do much besides sleeping.

Frances heard about the "Feeling Great!" program in the newspaper. She had never before participated in an exercise program but decided to give it a try. From the first day she loved the class, the activity and the fellow participants. She became a regular participant and never missed a class in two years. She always comes to class 45 minutes before it begins and stays to the very end of each session.

In class, Frances learned how to swim and became an avid swimmer. She also learned how to walk briskly and now walks a mile before each class session. After a year in the program she was able to walk briskly up to three miles. She is now always on the go and exclaims that she can jump onto the bus, whereas before she could barely get on. Before coming to the program, she always stayed home, but since she began participating in the program she is now a butterfly always on the go, shopping and browsing in stores.

One of the group members, Joyce, organized a five-day bus trip through the southeast states which Frances participated in. This was Frances' first vacation since she was a child. Frances was overjoyed taking the trip with her new friends at the "Feeling Great!" program. All during the trip she kept on telling Joyce that she must be sent by God to have organized such a beautiful trip for the class. Frances came back from the trip beaming like a new person, fresh, healthy, alive, full of vigor, and feeling rejuvenated.

Frances looks forward to coming to the program twice a week, meeting her friends, and getting her regular dose of exercise. At 77 years old she is one of the strongest, healthiest members of the class. Her vitality seems to come from her renewed faith in herself and feeling that she is healthy, feels great, and can still enjoy the many pleasures of life.

JOYCE DUSANG

Joyce was a very active person in her youth involved with swimming, tumbling, and playing sports. She worked a desk job as a quality control analyst for many years in New Orleans. She claims that due to her sedentary lifestyle in adulthood, her desk job, and the good food in New Orleans, she became overweight and out of shape. When Joyce took early retirement from work at age 63 she called the downtown YMCA to see if they had an exercise class suited to her needs. She had enjoyed the daily drive from the suburbs into the city to work and wanted to continue to come into the city on a regular basis after she retired. She felt it would help her psychologically, feeling active, to come downtown to exercise. She would also have a chance to periodically meet and have lunch with her old companions from work, and gave her access to other things in the city.

When Joyce came to the program she commented that she was surprised to find such a nice caliber of people with varying abilities and different interests. She was also happy to find out that she was able to do most of the exercises and to slowly tone up and develop within the program. Joyce became a social leader in the group, lightening up the class with her humor, discussions, and interests in others. Sometimes after class she would go to lunch with some class members or help out a disabled participant with shopping or other needs.

Joyce describes herself as a follower all of her life. But in the "Feeling Great!" program she became a leader. She organized a five-day bus tour of the southern states for participants in the "Feeling Great!" program and is planning a group trip to Las Vegas for the future. She always helps by offering suggestions for our bi-weekly trips or contributing to the special functions and parties at the program. She even had pens made up with her name and "Feeling Great!" "Lee Circle YMCA" printed on them to distribute to class members. With her free time Joyce has begun to volunteer at a local hospital as a receptionist. She has truly become a leader among her peers, seeking new opportunities and reaching out to help others.

Joyce finds the "Feeling Great!" program helpful in her physical

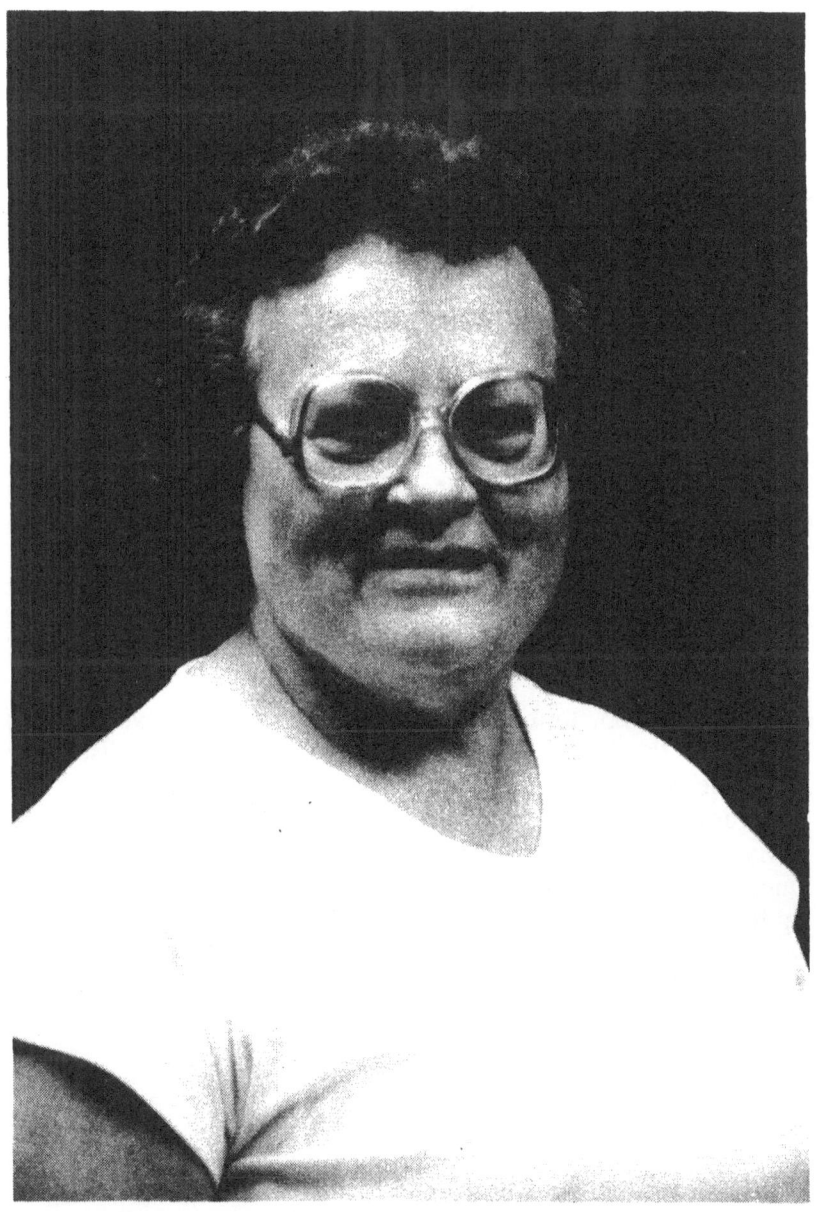

Joyce Dusang

fitness and also intellectually stimulating through the group health lectures and discussions. She shares the health care information and pamphlets she obtains from the class with neighbors and friends. Since she began the program she has shown improvement in flexibility and endurance and has begun to loose some weight and tone up.

Joyce greatly benefits from the "Feeling Great!" program because she is both a participant and leader in the group. A person who is willing to share, to learn, to bring new ideas and opportunities to others, and have fun with the group, Joyce has a very healthy attitude towards life. She always has a kind word and a smile for everyone, a person who makes you "Feel Great!"

MYRTLE AND URSULA HILL

Ursula Hill, age 63, joined the "Feeling Great!" program to help with her disabling arthritis, her limited leg movement due to a prosthesis in her knee, and for a social outlet. When Ursula first came to the program she walked with a cane and traveled over an hour by bus to come to class. After being in the group for a couple of months she proudly announced that her sister, Myrtle, would soon join the class.

Myrtle, age 55, took an early retirement from her work as the assistant to the supervisor of housing for the 8th Naval district in New Orleans. She retired to spend more time to help her sister and her bedridden, 93-year-old mother with their daily needs.

Myrtle and her sister never married and lived with their mother. Since Ursula was handicapped and didn't drive, Myrtle did the driving for the family and took on many of the chores and responsibilities around the home. Myrtle was a thin woman but in very good health which she credited to the hard work she did around the home, such as painting, fixing things, and taking care of the lawn and garden.

When Myrtle first came to the group she was quiet, but slowly blossomed into being more outgoing, very helpful to others and politely outspoken in her opinions. After only a few months in the program, Myrtle assisted new participants in learning the exercises and becoming acquainted with other group members. She would caution and jest with new members about my sometimes humorous

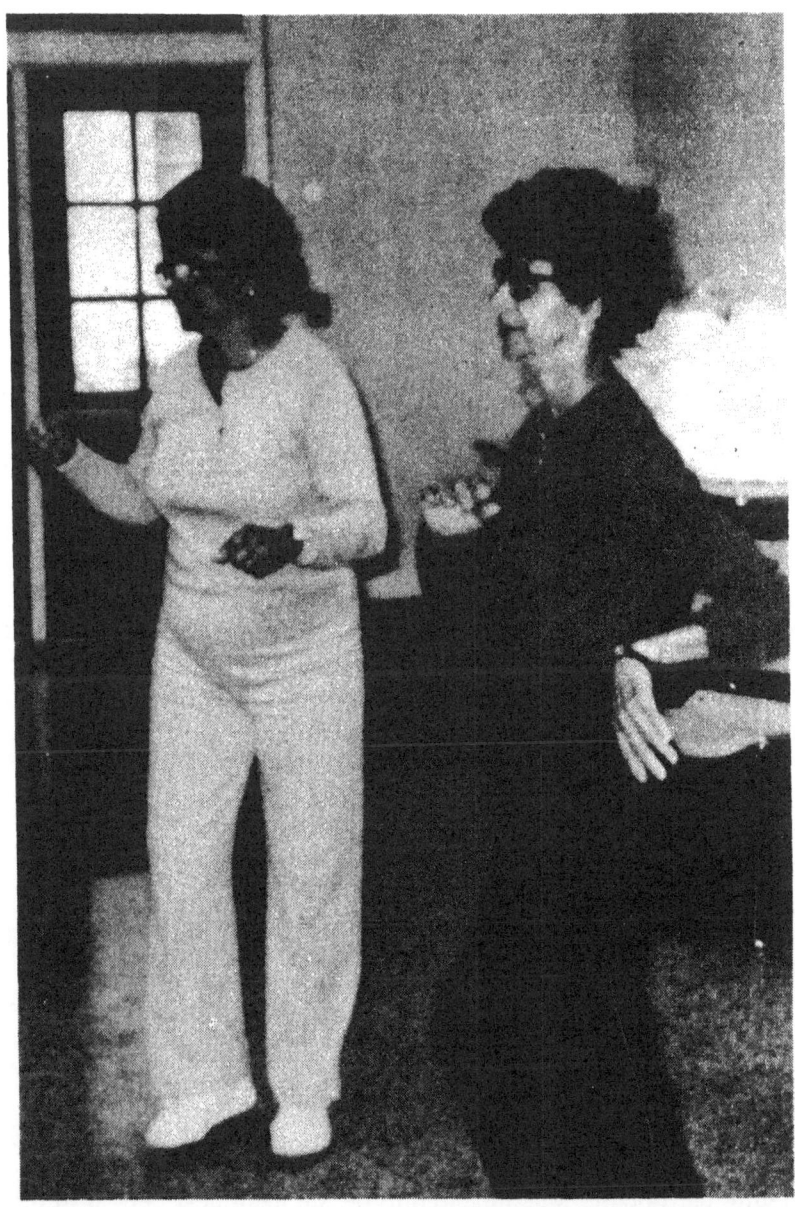

Myrtle and Ursula Hill—snapshot taken during a "Feeling Great!" class, 1986

and outrageous style of interacting with the class, which she enjoyed very much, giving her an emotional lift.

During the health lectures Myrtle seemed to benefit from the discussions on our "spiritual responsibility." I often talked about helping others, as reflected in the old Hebrew proverb from the Pirke Avot (known as Teachings of the Fathers): "If I am not for myself, who is for me? And if I am only for myself, what am I? And if not now, when?" True wellness is not a selfish narcissistic regime of exercising and dieting but rather a growing awareness of how best to take care of ourselves, to relate with others, and to be a positive influence and integral part of the world we touch.

Though financially supporting her sister and mother on a limited budget, Myrtle would routinely tithe to the church and volunteer to play the church organ at services. She also conducted the adult choir in her church. Through the many talks we had in our health lectures concerning the needs of the younger generation and our resources as older mature adults, Myrtle was inspired to develop a children's choir at her church. She had much success with the new choir. They sang weekly at the church and in the community at various holiday functions. Myrtle epitomized everything I taught; to take responsibility for and care of yourself, and to be a support and inspiration to others.

Whenever I was out of town, Myrtle would run the "Feeling Great!" class. I heard that she conducted the session like a loving navy sergeant. She was much more regimented than I, counting out each exercise activity to make sure everyone did the exercises together. Her health lectures were often group discussions of pertinent issues concerning older adults. She gave people a chance to talk and be heard.

On Thursday morning, March 5, 1987, before class, Ursula called me at the YMCA to say that Myrtle had just died. I said, "You mean your mother died." She said, "No, Myrtle died, she never woke up from her sleep." Myrtle died of a heart attack.

In class, Myrtle appeared as strong and well as I, though I was 20 years younger. On the day she died she was scheduled for a checkup with her doctor. She appeared to be the healthiest person in the "Feeling Great!" program, and had her doctor's permission to participate.

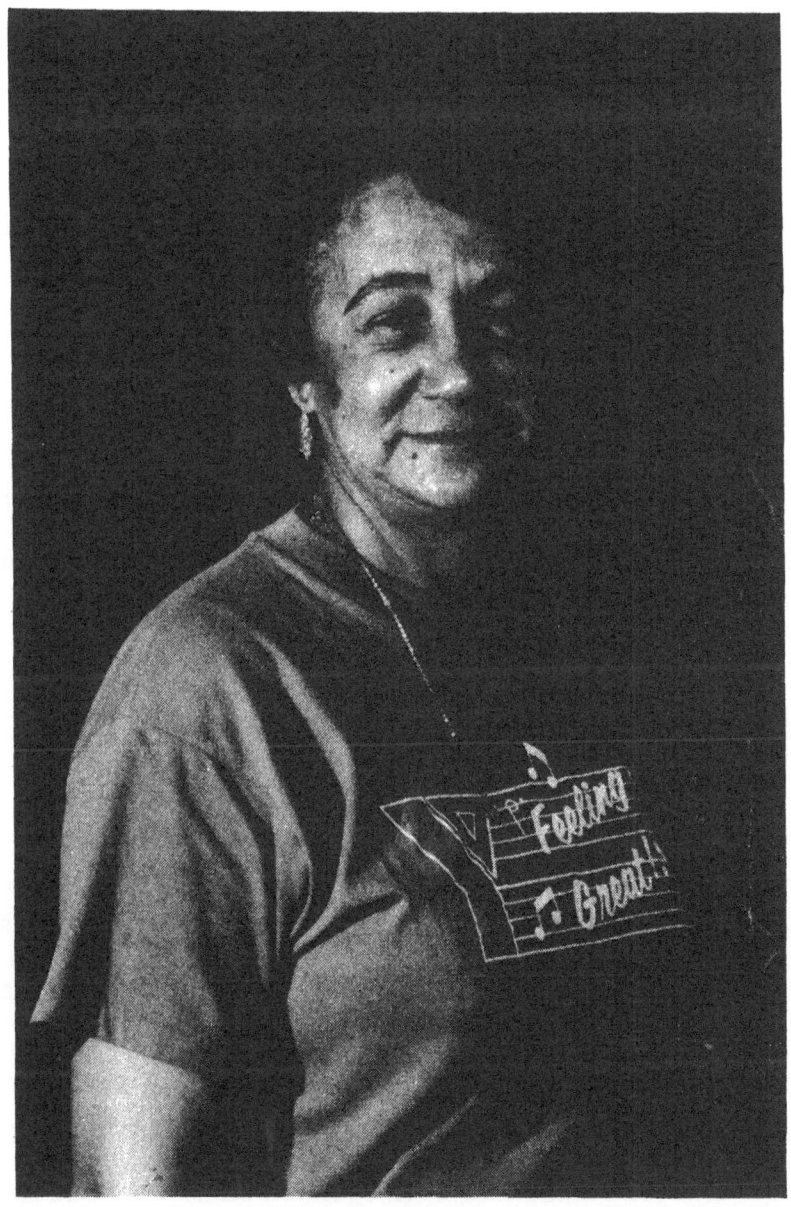

Ursula Hill, 1987

In the two years of the program's existence no participants had ever died. The greatest shock to the group was Myrtle's death. She had been the top participant and leader in the group. She was one of the only individuals in the group to have no arthritis and no disability. The group couldn't understand it. We have had so many other people join the group who were much older and more lacking in physical and mental health. We could only wonder why Myrtle, why her?

As an afternote, since Myrtle's death Ursula had the full charge of taking care of both her home and her bedridden mother. Ursula's sister, Lula, daily came over to take care of her mother. Ursula also obtained the assistance of an aide from a social service agency to help with her mother's care two days a week. Within six months of Myrtle's death, their mother died. Having both of her lifelong companions die within a year, Ursula, in coping with her grief and sorrow reached out to spend more time with her family and friends (including members of the "Feeling Great!" program) and continued to develop her independent life.

The "Feeling Great!" program has been Ursula's companion for over three years, witnessing and aiding her in the daily struggles, helping her to regain her physical health, and assisting her in coping with the death of her mother and sister.

OLGA JEFFERSON

Olga, age 81, is an active participant of the "Feeling Great!" program and attends class whenever she is not working. Though she suffers from severe arthritis pain she works on a regular basis as a sitter for people who are ill, thereby helping to support her extended family. She loves her work and is very committed to helping those who have difficulty helping themselves.

Olga has a wit and aliveness that you would expect a teenager to possess. In her subdued way she loves to tell stories, many funny, some risqué, and always seems to draw a crowd around her. She is very active in her church and senior citizen center "Golden Age" club, holding various positions of responsibility.

Her participation in the "Feeling Great!" program helps to keep

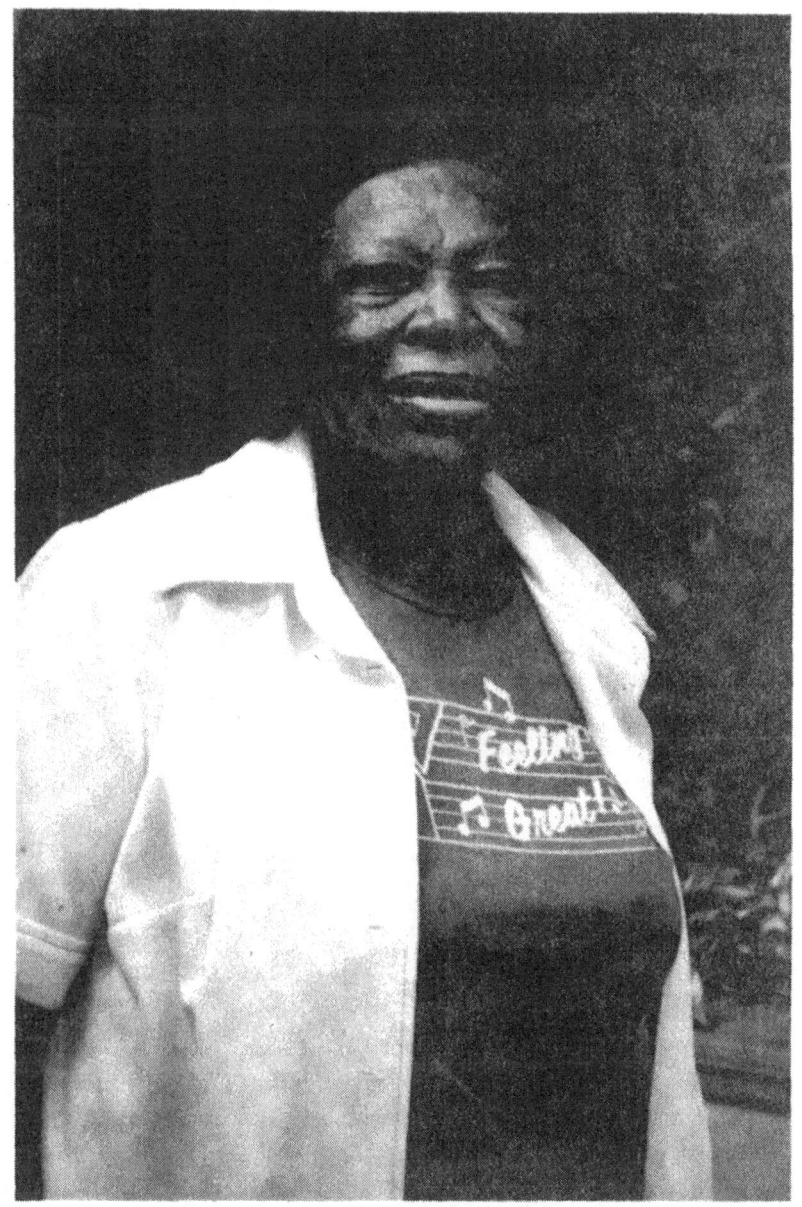

Olga Jefferson

her limber and reduces some of her arthritis pain. She loves the work-out, the health care lectures and the good company.

Olga is the type of person who is there when you need her; a person who knows how hard life can be and how wonderful it is. Besides her other talents she is a writer, speaker, and leader of her times.

Someone Who Cares

If you can't come to see me when I'm living,
why bother when I die?
Can't smile at you, shake your hand,
or say "How have you been?"
It only takes a second to write a little note.
If you're out of stamps
you can use the phone.
It's strange you're soon forgotten
as the years go passing by.
You wonder where old friends are.
I'll think I'll drop a line,
maybe they're sick or lonesome,
waiting for a call.
Relatives are getting fewer—
some have none at all.
Why not keep in touch with each other?
Let them know you care.
Tomorrow may be too late for a visit.
When you can, they won't be there.

Mrs. Olga Jefferson

GLORIA BATINICH

Joan saw an article in the newspaper about the "Feeling Great!" program and thought it would be wonderful for her mother, Gloria. Gloria had been homebound for seven months recovering from a leg injury and was grieving over the death of her other daughter due to cancer. She suffered from daily asthma attacks and had severe arthritis pain in her hands, shoulders, and knees. For Christmas of

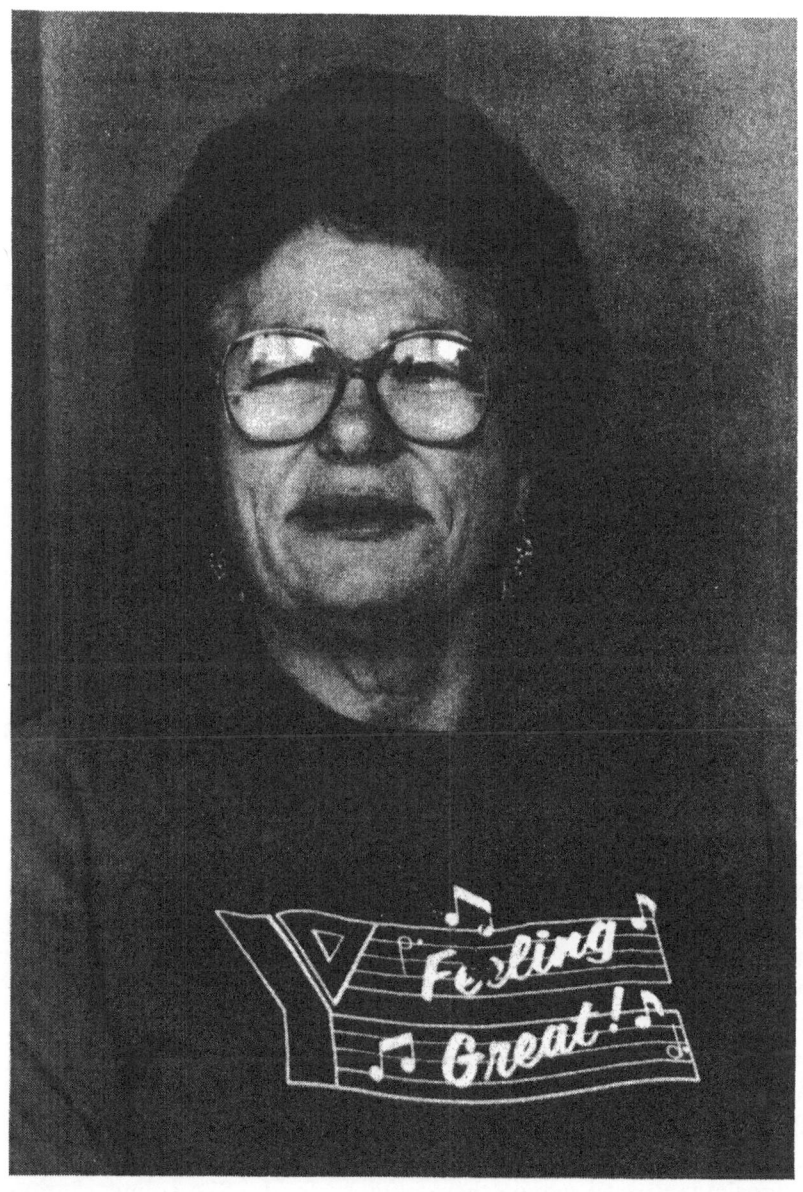

Gloria Batinich

1985, Joan gave her mother a six month gift certificate to the "Feeling Great!" program. At first, Gloria was hesitant about joining the program but soon fell in love with it.

Gloria was home alone for an extensive time due to her illness and had too much time on her hands which she spent worrying and grieving. As a result, she became more depressed and isolated. Joan knew that Gloria needed to exercise, to meet new people, and be motivated with some fresh ideas; Joan hoped that the "Feeling Great!" program would fill the social and physical health needs in her mother's life.

Since her consistent participation in the program over the past two years along with her home exercise program Gloria, at age 62, has seen some tremendous results. Her asthma attacks decreased by 70% and she now feels no arthritis pain in any part of her body. These benefits can be attributed to attending the "Feeling Great!" program twice a week, a *daily* exercise program consisting of walking in her neighborhood or at the park, and riding her exercise bicycle at home.

Though Gloria has accomplished much, her daughter told me that at times she still gets lazy and discouraged. At these times, Gloria needs motivation to exercise and attend the exercise class. But when Gloria comes home from class, her daughter observes that she has a better attitude about herself and life in general. She is like a new person! Gloria claims that the class discussions and health lectures help her to cope with daily difficulties and reinforces a healthy productive attitude in facing life. No matter what health or financial problems she faces she always says it could be worse, and there are other people who are not as fortunate as I, so I will be thankful for my situation in life. Now, Gloria has become a great motivator for others and contributes to the class with her new found sense of emotional and physical well-being.

Gloria was a quiet person when she joined the program but then blossomed and became a spark of joy in the class. Born in Yugoslavia, she often tells the group stories of her life in the "old country." She is also a good cook and for class parties she brings Yugoslavian pastries and other delicious foods. She enjoys sharing the happiness, troubles, and wisdom gained in her life and listens to others with empathy and concern. Whenever a participant needs a ride home after class, Gloria is always happy to take them. She is a very generous person in all ways.

Since we already had another person named Gloria in the class and wanted to keep everyone on a first name basis, I affectionately nicknamed her Yugo, after the Yugoslavian car, and call her my foreign exchange student. Sharing humor is a part of making each class new and alive. Gloria also makes a contribution in this area such as referring to the exercises as her "shake and bake" program. She has become an avid participant in the program and it has become a major part of her life. The "Feeling Great!" program is her support group, her extended family, a place where she can feel uplifted and let go of the troubles of the day. It provides a time and place for her to do something special for herself—exercising and socializing with friends.

Ultimately, the "Feeling Great!" program is shaped by the instructor and the participants and reflects their attitudes. New people joining the program find such a pleasant atmosphere which is due to having nice people like Gloria, who make it a success for all.

"FEELING GREAT!" PARTICIPANTS WERE ASKED "HOW HAS THE PROGRAM HELPED YOU?"

Frances, age 77—"It has increased my social life. Before I began the program I just stayed home and felt tired all of the time. But now I go out by myself to various stores and activities in the community. I seem to have so much more energy to do things."

Hattie, age 54—"I can walk much better now! A few years ago I had a stroke and suffered partial paralysis on the right side of my body. Walking was so difficult I got a wheelchair to get around. But, since I joined the program I do not even have to use my cane anymore. I can control my balance much better and have better use of my limbs."

Joyce, age 64—"When I was younger I was so much more active. After years of a desk job and a sedentary lifestyle I became overweight and out of shape. It feels great to become active again."

Margaret M., age 80—"I enjoy keeping in shape and the friendship I find in the group. I really like the discussions we have."

Margaret G., age 59 — "I take care of my 93-year-old father at home and I need to get out of the house for my own well-being, it's so stressful at times. When I come to the program I feel like a different person. I forget my troubles, enjoy the exercise and friendship, and get a chance to talk with my friends and share stories. It's so important for my mental health to come to the program!"

Gloria B., age 62 — "Since I began the program it seems that my arthritis pain has gone away. I also feel so much better since I began walking on a daily basis around my neighborhood. Our discussions at the program lift my spirits when I feel troubled. You know everyone has problems, but it's just how you deal with them and this program has helped me with my attitude toward my problems. Also it's a group I feel comfortable with and always feel better to be among."

Audry, age 61 — "I enjoy the group and it gives me a chance to exercise which I wouldn't do by myself. I also learned how to swim at the age of 61."

Delores, age 51 — "I use to be tired all of the time, now I seem to have more energy and I feel better about myself."

Evelyn, age 68 — "Before I came to the program my mother had just died and I was very depressed. The group support helped me during that time. I was also very scared of over exerting myself but now I just love the exercise and feel comfortable in our work-out session. I feel better than ever and I am in good health."

Elaine, age 53 — "I learned how to swim at the program. It goes to show you that at any age you can still learn new things. I also love the companionship. I used to be a television soap opera addict, but now I am so busy in my life I forgot about television. I also really enjoy volunteering in the program and doing my part in helping out by calling members who missed a class or are ill. It gives me a reason to call everyone periodically."

Mary, age 70+ — "Before I began the program I could not bend down to tie my shoes nor could I walk up and down the stairs without having a lot of pain. Now I can do both activities easily. I have much more flexibility in my body and can move around with very little arthritis pain."

Marie, age 70 — "After my stroke I joined the program and I feel a lot better since I joined. It has really helped my whole life. I've improved in my range of motion, leg strength, and arm and hand strength."

Abbie, age 69 — "I was wobbly when I walked and often lost my equilibrium. The program has helped me to be able to walk steadily, with ease and greater balance. I can also walk much faster now. I used to have chest pains often due to angina, but now I have them much less frequently."

Ida, age 71 — "After I retired I wanted to get active and it feels good to come to the group. I lost some weight by coming here. Now I sleep better and I feel better when I wake up in the morning. I enjoy the class, the people and the social aspect of the program. I especially like the field trips we take. My arms used to hurt, but since I have been exercising I have no pain. I also used to be afraid of the water but now I can swim the length of the pool and it feels great! I really enjoy the health lectures, the information, and our discussions, it is all very interesting."

Doris, age 85 — "I have improved my walking and gained better coordination. I also really enjoy being with my group of friends, who make me feel special. Whenever I have to miss class I really miss the socializing and I find that my body gets stiff."

Ursula, age 65 — "Participating in the program has really helped to improve my flexibility. Overall it's helped me emotionally through some difficult times and physically in my struggle with arthritis. I have made some wonderful new friends and I always enjoy coming to the program. I've also learned how to swim and it has really helped my arthritic condition."

Glory, age 70 — "It's a great activity and I look forward to being with the group. The program gives me incentive to lose weight. It also gives me a better attitude about myself and I really enjoy doing volunteer work for Jules."

Bridget, age 70 — "The program has given me an awareness of myself, my body and my feelings. I've made new friends and I really enjoy the field trips we take together."

Anna, age 54 — When asked the question, "How has the program helped you?" Anna insisted on taking a couple of days to think over her answer and to give it to me in writing as noted below.

Dec. 11, 1987

I noticed a marked increase in stamina, being able to stay active for a longer period during the day, and this was only after a few weeks. But in addition to this feeling of well-being, there were other benefits.

As a group, members in the "Feeling Great!" program are very supportive of each other and are interested in the well-being of their fellow members. The leader's encouragement, genuine concern and good humor not only lifts morale but has the effect of unifying its members.

Mr. Weiss' informal discussions on diet, exercise, and current health issues kept these matters on the frontline and made me aware personally of the importance of good health maintenance. Each "Feeling Great!" member shared their experiences and we felt free to express our opinions — in short, we could be "ourselves."

A lot of credit is due Mr. Weiss' sensitive leadership. He's a man with a special talent for helping others. He helps us not only to feel good physically, but to feel good about ourselves and then, taking with us his words of encouragement, we leave the "Feeling Great!" group with confidence to go out to help our family and friends, like an ever-widening circle.

Anna Tuminello

Sylvia, age 52 — When I asked Sylvia how the program has helped her and her mother (who is also a participant of the program), Sylvia insisted on writing about it. In fact within a week she gave me three two page letters on how the program has helped her and her mother. I have reprinted her most recent letter on the program.

Jan. 5, 1988

To Whom It May Concern and To All Who Are Interested:

The "Feeling Great!" program at the YMCA has really been beneficial to my mom and me. Like many elderly people my mom, age 75, suffered from grief and loneliness along with severe depression since her husband passed away. With the doctor's care and of course the support of my family, I have continually tried to motivate her. The doctor had said that she came a long way from her previous depression and physical illness and my efforts were not in vain. Three years ago she was a candidate for lifetime institutionalization because she could not take care of herself and she gave up her desire to live. But, as her daughter, I accepted this challenge with love and tried to help motivate her and keep her active.

The "Feeling Great!" class is an answer from god for my mom. This class has helped her to realize that she is a youthful elderly person and she has made many new friends. The exercises have been beneficial to the degree of increasing her circulation, making her more alert and active, and now she can even stay up till 9:00 p.m. whereas before she went to bed at 5:00 p.m. She also has a happier outlook on life since she began the program and always looks forward to attending the class. Before she had nothing to look forward to.

My hands are full considering I am also a wife and mother to three children. However thankful I am to God for the added years of my mother's life, I would not be truthful if I did not say that taking care of her has brought extra stress upon me. I have been able to cope, but unfortunately the way I used to cope was to eat more during the day and I became obese. So, I also need the "Feeling Great!" program to help me learn how to cope better with my stress. The emotional support which the class provides uplifts my spirits and helps me to cope with my stress. The swimming part of the program really helps me to unwind and relieves my tension. Also, since I joined the program I've been motivated to diet and have lost 6 pounds.

Mr. Jules Weiss shows strength in many areas as an individual and most certainly deserves recognition and congratulations as he is a great instructor and teacher with compassion and divine love that flows to meet each individual's needs no matter their health problem, handicap, age, weight, stress, etc.

His personality is dynamic and his charisma flows like a

river to each person. His sense of humor livens up the group and brings unity and harmony within the group. The end result in class is that everybody forgets their age, their many problems, their loneliness, and other difficulties. They smile, talk and joke with one another, and are happy which produces a unity and sharing among the group.

His concern for those who are absent due to illness or are out of town is ever present. His interesting health lectures are simplified and easy to comprehend. You can hear a pin drop during the lecture but yet we are eager to ask questions and discuss the lecture material.

"Feeling Great!" in '88 is an asset to us and we share the good news of what has happened to us and is available for you.

Sincerely,
Sylvia LeBlanc

P.S. Mr. Jules Weiss has shown with his busy schedule of wife, children, writing, counseling and jobs that his attitude never changes and he is eager to help us stay physically fit and well. He is a positive thinker who sets his goals and doesn't look back which makes him so successful and inspiring to us in reaching our goals. He is a great teacher and a great leader. He tries to always do what is best for others without imposing his will on them. Many thanks to you Mr. Weiss for helping me and so many others in a similar situation. We appreciate you!

Chapter III

Program Mechanics

BARRIERS TO PARTICIPATION

The barriers and difficulties for older adults in participating in exercise classes cover a wide spectrum of social, psychological, and physical issues. The many normal fears and apprehensions some senior citizens may have of exercising and joining a new program can easily deter them. For this reason, it is imperative that the exercise instructor conscientiously address the possible problems and fears older adults may face when entering a new exercise/health education program. Listed below are some barriers to participation which are subcategorized into three areas: *Psychological*, *Social*, and *Physical*.

A. Psychological

1. Depression
2. Fear of embarrassment
3. Lack of confidence in their ability to do the exercises
4. Lack of motivation or too easily discouraged
5. Afraid that the instructor will ask them to exercise more than they are able to
6. Afraid that the exercises will be too strenuous
7. Afraid that they do not have the correct clothes to exercise in
8. Conditioned to believe they need to slow down and not be as active

B. Social

1. Feel uncomfortable coming to the program without a friend or not knowing anyone

2. Feel embarrassed about being out of shape or overweight
3. Feel self-conscious about possibly not being able to keep up with the class
4. Afraid of what their friends and family may think
5. Prospective male participants may think this type of program is only for women, or if the group is primarily composed of women, men may feel out of place (and vice versa for women).
6. Afraid of leaving the safety of their home to go to a community based program
7. Feel the program costs more than they can afford

C. Physical

1. Out of shape and ashamed about the condition of their body and their lack of strength, balance and/or stamina
2. Afraid of hurting themselves by exercising
3. Afraid the exercises will be too strenuous

SPECIFIC DETERRENTS AND REMEDIES

There are some specific deterrents participants may find to joining or continuing their participation in an exercise program. These deterrents may be overcome with careful planning, proper facility coordination, clear supportive communication with participants and fellow staff, and flexibility within the program. Listed below are a few common deterrents and possible remedies.

1. *Deterrent* — Transportation
   Remedy — Provide bus schedules, help organize car pools, or contract with a private van service.
2. *Deterrent* — Parking
   Remedy — Provide a list of convenient parking places and/or arrange with a garage to offer low cost parking.
3. *Deterrent* — Class is too expensive
   Remedy — Offer reduced rates for those people who cannot afford the full price. Ask the participants, in compensation for a free reduction, if they would like to help out with the program by volunteering their services.

4. *Deterrent* — Fear of looking ugly in shorts
   Remedy — Impress upon participants that this is a closed group and they will be among their peers who probably do not look much different. Participants can wear stretch pants or jogging suits.
5. *Deterrent* — Participants fear that the exercises will be too fast a pace or too strenuous for them to keep up.
   Remedy — Make special provisions to allow participants to go at their own pace (slower or faster), stress the importance of exercising at a comfortable rate; it's not how good you look, it's how great you feel!
6. *Deterrent* — Feeling too out of shape for the class
   Remedy — Explain that the class is designed for people who are out of shape or who have not exercised in a while. The sessions are geared to help people to slowly tone up and get into better shape.
7. *Deterrent* — Depression
   Remedy — Explain that at times it may be difficult for participants to feel motivated to attend class, but usually they will feel much better after coming to the class. The class can help take their mind off negative and depressing thoughts, and improve their outlook on life.
8. *Deterrent* — Some people are "turned off" by the word exercise.
   Remedy — In describing the program you can use the word activity instead of exercise: physical, muscular, or aerobic activity.
9. *Deterrent* — Only male or female participants in the class, so participants of the other sex may hesitate to join
   Remedy — Stress that the class is both for males and females, and encourage the minority sex in the class to attend by giving them some special class attention. Also, it may help to offer a class special such as, if they bring a friend his/her first class is free and the group member gets one free class.
10. *Deterrent* — Participants fear that they may have to do something in the class that they do not want to do.
    Remedy — Explain that all activities are voluntary and the class members understand that some participants will not be able to

do certain exercises due to physical problems. Try to make the program as pleasant and stress-free as possible because, if the participants do not enjoy the program, they probably will not continue coming to the class.

11. *Deterrent*—Fear of being a failure in class
    Remedy—Explain that this is a noncompetitive learning class. Each person exercises according to his or her abilities and limitations. No one is critical of what a person can or cannot do, we only encourage people to try to do the best they can.

12. *Deterrent*—Class members competing with each other
    Remedy—Make sure you praise everyone for their efforts no matter what their ability, downplay any competition, and be careful of participants who show off. At times showing off can be a good ego boost, but it also can make participants very self-conscious. The instructor should adjust the activities to keep the competitive aspects of the activity limited to having fun rather than showing off or out-doing each other.

13. *Deterrent*—class members who continually complain about their physical ailments and problems
    Remedy—Accept participants' complaints, do not deny their feelings but point out the positive aspects of their life and how they can develop better health and fitness. Explain to the group the ill effects a negative attitude can have and show how a positive approach to life is most helpful. A negative attitude does not help anyone, it only hinders.

THE INTERACTION OF MEDICATION, NUTRITION, AND EXERCISE

The interaction of medication, nutrition, and exercise can aid a person in having outstanding health or produce detrimental effects depending on the circumstances.* For example, food and exercise can enhance, delay, or decrease the absorption of medication.

---

*Some of the noted material is adapted from the article "The Interactionary Effects of Medication, Nutrition, and Exercise" by C.J. Jones, PhD in *The Southwestern, The Journal Of Aging For The Southwest*. Vol 3, 1986, p. 57-74.

Effects of Medications on Food

1. Medications can alter the taste or smell of certain foods, such as making them taste bland, causing the individual to lose interest in eating.
2. Medications may increase or decrease a person's appetite.
3. Medications can induce feelings of nausea or cause sores or inflammation of the mouth.
4. Certain medications can change the absorption rate of particular food nutrients whereas people taking certain drugs may need a vitamin supplement.
5. Individuals who take prescriptive medicines for chronic conditions over a long period of time can become more vulnerable to malnutrition due to the drugs' effects on their body as noted above. Some other possible ill effects of medications are:

   a. inactivation of enzymes necessary for absorption of minerals;
   b. increased renal excretion;
   c. decreased intestinal absorption of nutrients.

Effects of Medications on the Body

1. Certain medications like Darvocet can make people feel tired while others such as amphetamines can cause them to feel they have a lot of energy, regardless of the physical condition of their bodies. These drugs can give people a false feeling about the state of their body's condition and vital signs, i.e., heart rate, blood pressure, thus individuals should carefully monitor their vital signs during the exercise activity.
2. Though exercise conducted in a program that progressively helps a person to tone up is known to help reduce high blood pressure, for people taking high blood pressure medication strenuous exercise can be very hazardous. Strenuous exercise, especially isometric exercises and heavy weightlifting can increase participants' blood pressure while their medication is trying to decrease the blood pressure. Individuals who take medication for high blood pressure should focus on flexibility and light aerobic exercises to slowly build up their cardiovascular system.

3. Some people take diuretic drugs for high blood pressure/hypertension to reduce their body fluid and relax their arteries in order to lower blood pressure and muscle tension. A possible adverse reaction of this drug with exercise is dehydration. It is essential that exercise leaders reinforce to those participants who are taking diuretics to drink plenty of fluids during and after exercising.
4. For some older adults, due to the need to take many medications, adverse reactions can be caused by the mixing of various drugs.
5. Poor compliance in a person's medication regime or being over-medicated due to confusion over which pills to take can cause very serious problems.

Effects of Foods on Medication

1. Certain foods can alter the absorption and excretion rate of particular drugs in a person's body. Inevitably, this can cause certain medications to stay in the body longer than expected which over time can result in a toxic effect to the individual. Older adults who take many medications for chronic conditions over an extended length of time are more susceptible to this problem.
2. Certain foods should not be taken with particular drugs due to the drug/food interaction in the body which can neutralize the effects of the medication. Tetracycline is such a drug, which cannot be taken with milk, milk products, or antacids. Another example is tobacco and caffeine which will decrease the effect of nitroglycerin.
3. Many older adults, at times, have trouble motivating themselves to eat properly. Some of their eating problems stem from:

   • the food has a lack of taste and smell due to the side effects of certain medications or due to the physical aging process of the individual's body;
   • apathy in eating due to the loneliness of cooking and eating alone;
   • depression;
   • people who do not have teeth or who have poorly fitted dentures may find it difficult to eat.

   If older adults have a lack of appetite over an extended period of time and begin to greatly reduce their diet, then their medications may not become absorbed at the rate they were prescribed for, or be as effective in the body.

The Body's Need for Water

Often older adults do not think they are thirsty even when their bodies may need a drink. This is because their thirst mechanism often lags behind their actual level of dehydration. It is vital that possibly during and definitely after exercising each person has a drink of water or other fluids. This will prevent dehydration and provide the needed sufficient liquids to compensate for lost fluids during exercise.

Effects of Exercise

1. For people with high blood pressure/hypertension, isometric and heavy weight lifting exercises should be avoided. These exercises can cause the blood to build up too much force through the vascular system. While exercising, it is most important for participants to be able to comfortably breathe without needing to gasp for a breath. Breathing aids in circulation.
2. For participants who have high blood pressure/hypertension, the monitoring of their heart rate is very important during the exercise session to monitor the work intensity on their heart.
3. For diabetics exercising on a regular basis can help to increase insulin efficiency by increasing the number of insulin receptors on muscle cells. This is especially true of endurance type exercises such as brisk walking, and swimming. While exercising, sugar is removed from the blood stream to supply the muscles, and liver production of glucose from stored glucose is stopped, thus further lowering the blood sugar. Careful regulation of exercise duration and intensity, medication, and diet is extremely important and should be monitored and reported by participants to their physician.
4. Exercising for arthritis is very effective, especially flexibility exercises which help to increase the range of motion of joints. Exercise can help to improve circulation problems associated with arthritis and the pain and stiffness in the joints. Exercise instructors need to be alert to when, in certain cases, individuals' tissue

masses around joints are swollen due to arthritis and may become more aggravated by exercise. In these cases, participants should only lightly exercise excessively swollen joints.

Recommended Safety Warning to All Older Adults

It is essential to have participants' medications reviewed by a doctor every six months, especially if there has been a change in their diet or exercise routine. Older adults taking medications should ask their doctor or pharmacist the following questions:

- Do they need a vitamin supplement or to alter their diet?
- Should they drink a lot of water with the prescription?
- Will drinking alcohol affect the medication?
- What foods or drinks should they abstain from?
- If they exercise will it have an effect on the medication?
- Are there any possible adverse effects of the medication?

A word to the wise older adult: Be safe, be informed, and be cautious about exercise, medications, and good nutrition.

MOTIVATION

Motivation is a key to making a wellness and/or exercise program succeed for an individual. Motivation can be intrinsic to an individual's personality due to his/her background or it can be impressed upon a person (extrinsic motivation). Group support and the facilitator's approach can aid an individual's motivation, making the extrinsic process an intrinsic one through encouragement, peer support, and guidance.

It is advisable to have participants begin with small short-term goals that can be easily reached such as coming to the exercise program regularly, losing one or two pounds in a couple of weeks, or limiting the amount of sweets a person eats during the day. After participants experience success in some short-term goals they should then work up to striving for more long-term, personally desired goals.

WAYS TO INSTILL MOTIVATION

Sharing

1. Let participants inform the group about the improvements they have felt since coming to the program.
2. Provide a list of phone numbers of classmates so participants can call each other. Encourage participants to set up a "buddy system" and call each other to check if they are following a healthy diet, exercising daily, and to give each other emotional support. Encourage socialization outside of the program.
3. Provide time in the group for participants to tell about new exercises they are doing, positive changes in their diet, health tips, favorite nutritious recipes, and other interests.
4. Have participants tell about the positive remarks they received from family and friends since they began the program and the positive changes they have experienced.
5. Have group discussions during the health lecture segment of the class on issues and concerns facing older adults such as crime, family problems, assertiveness, etc.
6. Have one member be a volunteer in charge of sending out get-well cards to ill participants.
7. Have another volunteer call up members who have missed class to remind and encourage them to attend the next session. Also, have the volunteer inform them of the upcoming field trips.
8. Have participants discuss their progress in meeting their designated goals, as noted on the contract/goals and goals/homework/periodic review form, see page 180.
9. Participants can shape the program to their needs through their feedback to the instructor and by their volunteer efforts. Offering participants to take some responsibility in the success and progress of the program allows them to feel some ownership in the program as a contributing member.

Encouraging

1. Praise participants for their efforts. Give encouragement noting any small or large change you see participants achieve, be it in physical appearance, attitude, exercising ability or a number of

Holiday celebration

other areas. At times, an encouraging thought, personal recognition, and possibly some levity can lift the spirits of a discouraged participant.
2. Allow participants to shine in their own way. Show-off the positive aspects of class members' participation in the program.
3. For those people who show significant improvement, give verbal recognition and point out to others how they can also be helped by continuing the program and exercising at home.
4. In each class focus on several different people, complimenting on their activities and showing them how they can still improve their performance. A little personal attention and recognition is usually what people need and want. Sometimes it only takes a couple of positive sentences about the individual in front of the group to make the person feel important and good about his/her participation.

Activities

1. Give exercise and nutrition homework — exercises to do at home or a diet to reduce the intake of certain foods. Have participants tell the group how they keep to their exercise and nutrition homework plan and the difference it makes.
2. It may be helpful to do the following visualization activity in aiding participants to reach their personal fitness goals. Have participants visualize themselves reaching their goals and then tell each other how it feels once they have reached their goal. Remind participants that since they have already reached their goals in their mind, it only takes time, determination, and some work to physically reach their goals.
3. Provide rewards such as a free class, a certificate, or a tee-shirt with the class logo for significant gains such as consistent attendance for a month or for losing five pounds and keeping it off for a month.
4. After the group, participants can meet at a nearby restaurant for refreshments, snacks, or lunch and to socialize. Some restaurants will give a discount to senior citizen groups. Another option is to have participants bring snacks and make coffee or tea at the program while socializing during a break or after class. A

major component of the program is making new friends, interacting with peers, and having a good time.
5. Plan group outings at the end of an exercise session. It may be
best to keep the outings short between the hours of 11:30 a.m.
and 3:00 p.m. since the participants have spent a good deal of
time already exercising. Have the participants choose where they
want to go, whether it is to a cultural, recreational, sports or
dining activity.

HUMOR

I often use humor as a motivating tool in the "Feeling Great!"
program. Many participants feel apprehensive about exercising.
Joking can ease the tension and make them feel more relaxed in the
group setting. Humor can also be used for a variety of other reasons
such as:

- to enable participants to momentarily forget their aches, pains,
  and worries so they can interact and exercise freely;
- to stimulate new ideas and group interaction;
- to lose the sense of formality so participants can share their
  feelings and experiences more easily and be relaxed enough
  with each other to joke in a friendly manner;
- to help participants feel comfortable discussing topics they
  may be embarrassed mentioning such as sex, drugs, alcohol,
  family problems;
- to dissolve some erroneous assumptions such as senior citizens
  not having sexual or angry feelings;
- to promote unconditional acceptance and give a positive personal recognition to each participant regardless of his/her ability or attitude;
- to dissolve the emotional distance between participants and
  with the instructor and help them address each other as peers;
  and
- to acknowledge the difficulties people may face without embarrassing them.

The use of humor can create an almost euphoric feeling among the group, enabling participants to momentarily forget about their problems. At times, they can laugh with ease about the difficulties they face which lends to group support. Also, group members enjoy sharing jokes and amusing stories. One of the participants in the program who has a problem with depression claims that the laughter and joking in class help her to cope. At the end of class she does not feel depressed but rather invigorated for the rest of the day and can look back and laugh about the things that were said in group. Class members comment that joking lifts their spirits.

The use of humor is an art. To use it appropriately within a group setting it must not sound condescending, biased, negative, contrived, controlling or offensive. Humor can be provocative without offending. Humor must be used in a way that is supportive and sensitive to participants, providing positive attention and allowing them to build upon their interaction in a friendly creative manner. Humor should be spontaneous and joyous, lighting up the group spirit.

The use of humor can be healthy and productive in the group setting. Instructors must understand the effect humor has on the group process and activity and be able to change the group's conversational direction when needed.

The purpose of using humor is to enliven the group process. Joking in an exercise class is a sensitive matter and should be handled in a delicate way. Instructors can be "showmen/women" but not at the expense of the group or any individual. Instructors should always use good judgement on how, when, and why they use the tool of humor.

ATTITUDE GUIDELINES

A good, positive attitude is essential in providing a quality professional program. Noted below are some valuable guidelines which the instructor should be aware of while conducting the program.

1. If the instructor enjoys the class and is considerate of the participants, they will enjoy it also. Everyone wants to have a good
   time.
2. Be friendly, exuberant, it's contagious and personable.
3. Provide unconditional acceptance for participants' physical,
   emotional, and attitudinal situation. Have members share with
   the group the positive feedback they have gotten from family,
   friends, and group members since they began the program.
   Also, if they had gotten ridiculed for joining the program allow
   them to express their feelings and encourage the group to be a
   support for them. For participants who are afraid of trying new
   activities discuss the need for self-acceptance and permission to
   explore new areas. Help participants to make positive changes
   in their lives as they undertake new opportunities.
4. Be aware of participants' fears, limitations, and when they feel
   embarrassed in class.
5. Make the class a no-fail, noncompetitive experience for all.
6. Use humor and touching as a way to encourage participants to
   be informal, friendly, and relaxed. Let everyone interact on a
   first name basis.
7. At times it is healthy to be intimate with the class. If you share
   your fears and loves, they may do the same. Allow people to
   express their real feelings, so they can possibly deal with the
   real issues that prevent them from getting in better shape and
   health. A common fear may be the notion that they cannot
   achieve fitness or are unable to be in good shape and/or health.
   It can be said that staying fit is 40% exercise and 60% willpower. Without the willpower or motivation, people will not
   exercise. Remember, occasional exercise will only provide occasional benefit. But regular exercise will produce long-lasting
   cumulative effects. Encourage participants to exercise daily or
   every other day. Give exercise and diet homework.
8. Be kind and gentle. At some time you may have similar problems and attitudes especially if you have similar experiences.
9. While conducting the program be a teacher, listener, and student with participants. The more you work with participants
   and develop the program, the more you will learn how best you

can help them to make significant changes and gains in their lives.

10. Do not treat class members as children, and do not think that they are fragile because they are old. It is true that for some people their body is more fragile and probably out of shape, but they are adults with much experience and should be treated as such.

11. Know when to lend a hand and when you are crippling a person by helping them too much. People often do not need as much help as they need encouragement. Do not think you are helping people when you only do for them. "Feeling Great!" is a teaching and practicing class. You help people more by teaching them how to help themselves.

12. Do not talk down to anyone and be polite when correcting a person who may be doing an exercise the wrong way. One of the biggest mistakes for an exercise instructor is to embarrass a member of the class. Participants already often feel apprehensive about trying to get in shape. If you embarrass one person, others may think that they can be next so they may choose to drop out of the program in fear of being embarrassed.

13. One method of approaching individuals who are not exercising correctly is to address the whole group "on this common mistake" so no one is singled out or feels embarrassed in front of their peers.

14. Maintain an air of enthusiasm and encouragement about the effort each person makes in the class. It is better to praise a little effort and give encouragement than to tell participants what they are not doing or what they should be doing in a scolding manner.

15. The health lectures can be a very informative and vital service to the participants. Make the most of having the opportunity to teach preventive health care to the class.

16. The "Feeling Great!" class may be the most important thing in the participants' lives. It can provide them with a great amount of help, physically, emotionally, and socially. So conduct each class as though their lives depend upon it—because they do!

The program is as good as the instructor makes it!

STAFFING

A good staff person should be interested in the health and well-being of older adults. They should not be afraid of dealing with possibly depressing, conflictual, or difficult issues facing older adults when they arise. Furthermore, they should be energetic, excited, and committed to the program and its members.

Staff Personnel

1. primary staff person
2. assistant who may also act as a swimming instructor
3. optional swimming instructor if the assistant or primary staff person cannot teach swimming and water exercises

Staff Requirements

1. All staff should have some experience in working with adults and senior citizens.
2. All staff should understand that their primary concern is in furthering the independence, health, education, self-improvement, and wellness (physical fitness + health) of adults and senior citizens.
3. All staff will serve as educational, fitness, and motivational leaders for participants.
4. All staff should have the following certifications and fulfill the noted requirements:

   a. The YMCA basic fitness leadership certification
   b. C.P.R. and first aid certification from the Red Cross

5. Optional certifications which enhance the "Feeling Great!" program.

   a. "The Y's Way To A Healthy Back"
   b. "The Y's Way To Weight Management"
   c. "The Y's Way To Stress Management"
   d. Water exercise certification through the YMCA/Arthritis Foundation instructors' course

6. The swimming instructor should be certified as a YMCA lifeguard and instructor.

Suggested Staff Hours

Two days a week program:
Primary staff person — 15 hours a week
Assistant — 6 hours a week
Optional swimming instructor — 2 hours a week

Three days a week program:
Primary staff person — 20 hours a week
Assistant — 9 hours a week
Optional swimming instructor — 3 hours a week

Four or five days a week program:
Primary staff person — 30 hours a week
Assistant — 15 hours a week
Optional swimming instructor — 4 to 5 hours a week

Staff Schedule on Days Classes Are Held

Primary staff person — direct time — 8:00 a.m. to 2:00 p.m. — five hours, includes time for paperwork and field trips.

Assistant — direct time — 8:30 a.m. to 11:30 a.m. — three hours. It is preferable for this person to also assist in the pool to teach swimming and water exercises.

Optional swimming teacher — direct time — 10:30 a.m. to 11:30 a.m. — one hour. A swimming instructor will be needed if the assistant or primary staff person cannot aid in the pool while the other staff member directs the games, mat exercises, and relaxation session. A lifeguard should always be on duty with the swimming instructor during class time.

Exercise Class Schedule

The class should be held three times a week. It can be conducted effectively twice a week provided that participants practice their exercises at home to obtain the full benefit of the program.

Preferable Class Hours/Times

Tuesday-Thursday-Saturday
or *Monday-Wednesday-Friday*
Morning (e.g., 9:00 a.m.) is an excellent time for the class. Many older people get up very early in the morning. Classes after 5:00 p.m. are very good for working people. A Saturday morning class is usually good for most working people and for those who are retired or not employed.

VOLUNTEER INVOLVEMENT

Volunteers are an integral part of the "Feeling Great!" program. It would be wonderful if the program was conducted by senior citizens: Seniors teaching Seniors; Seniors as advocates for Seniors. Senior citizen staff and volunteers make the program more inviting to new members. Peer support, peer guidance, and peer relationships makes the program most effective.

All volunteers should be certified in first aid and C.P.R.

Volunteer Opportunities

1. *Participant Caller*—Duties: The day before class call participants who have missed the previous class to remind and encourage them to attend the next class and the next field trip. This volunteer would also be the representative from the group in charge of sending out get-well cards to those individuals who are ill.
2. *Organizer*—Duties: To set up the water jug and cups before every class along with setting out the exercise equipment. After class the volunteer would put everything away and make sure the exercise room is clean.
3. *Assistant Exercise Instructor*—Duties: When the regular exercise instructor is not able to conduct the class, the volunteer would conduct the exercise and health education portion of the program. The volunteer would be in charge of picking out the music to exercise with and researches and presents the health lecture. The volunteer instructor should be a participant of the

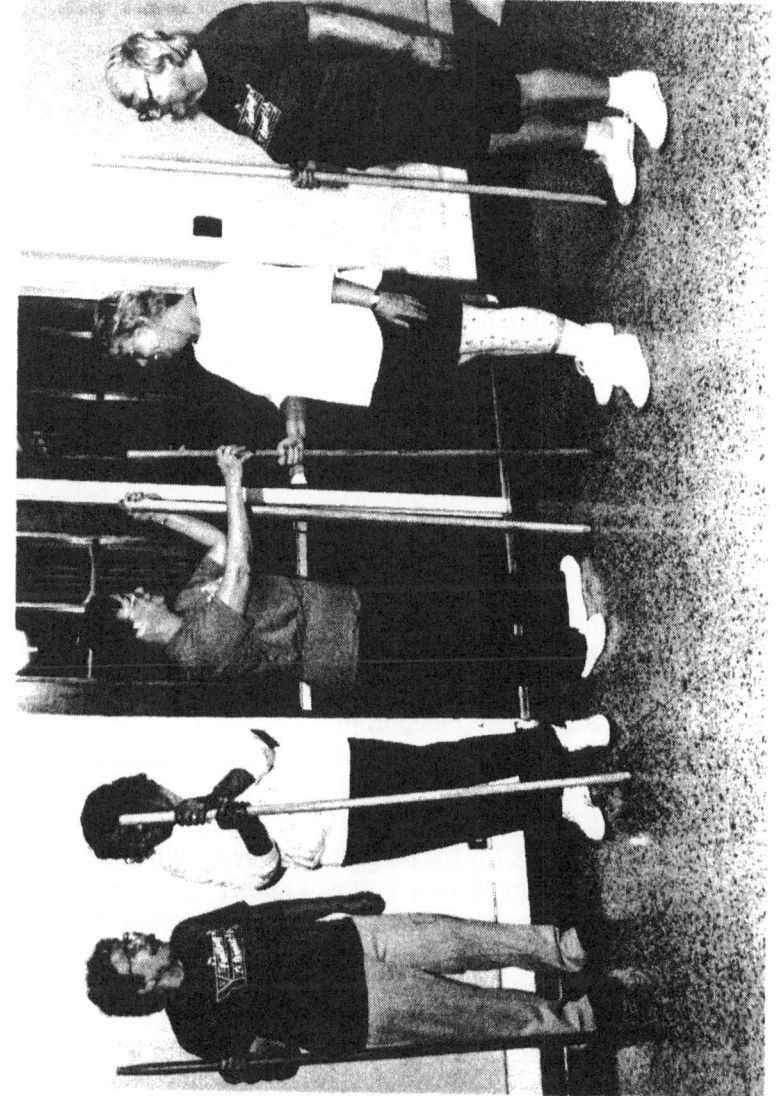

Volunteering – handing out the broomstick exercise equipment

program for at least six months, be in good physical condition, and exhibit mastery of all program activities.

4. *Assistant Swimming Instructor* — Duties: When the regular swimming instructor is not able to conduct the class, the volunteer would conduct the swimming/water exercise portion of the class. The volunteer must be able to teach participants how to swim along with knowing how to do water exercises. As previously noted, a lifeguard should always be on duty with the swimming instructor for safety precautions.

5. *Aide* — Duties: At the beginning of the class, the aide waits for new participants and directs them to the class. The aide orients new participants to the program by handing out brochures, program materials, and assists them with any questions or needs they may have. The aide may occasionally help participants in the dressing room.

FEES

The cost of the class may vary depending on the number of participants, space, and staff.

Suggested prices — $3.00 for one class, $5.00 for two classes per week, or for a shorter class session without swimming or water exercise $1.50 to $2.00 may be appropriate.

Prices should be set at a low cost to keep the class affordable to many older people who live on a fixed income. For those who cannot afford the class it is recommended that they pay a reduced rate and/or become volunteers for the program and be admitted for free. The program is not designed as a "money maker" but rather as a good comprehensive exercise/health education program and resource to meet the needs of people over the age of fifty.

For those participants who cannot afford the program it may be possible to obtain sponsors to finance their class sessions. Sponsors can contribute to the cost of the program for one or more participants monthly, every 6 months, or yearly. Possible sponsors are participants' family members, corporations, foundations, students, and the general public.

Corporations or agencies which allocate grants may either sponsor participants or subsidize the partial or complete cost of the program, enabling participants to join for free or at a reduced rate.

LIABILITY

If we could assure ourselves, and those who participate in exercise programs, that there is no risk or danger involved, we would have no need for any type of insurance coverage — liability, health, or accident. But, unfortunately accidents can happen and proper insurance coverage is necessary.

Before beginning an exercise program, it is important to find out if the facility is covered for liability and also if the exercise instructor is covered. Sometimes a person must be an employee of a facility to be covered under their liability insurance. An exercise instructor who is not an employee of the facility but rather a contractual employee may need his/her own coverage. A volunteer exercise instructor may also not be automatically covered by the facility's liability insurance plan. If requested, often the contractual or volunteer exercise instructor can be covered under the facility's insurance plan.

Accident Prevention Tips and Reporting

1. It is helpful for each participant to have a note from their doctor stating that they can participate in the program. Also, in case of an emergency participants should list the phone number of a person to contact and which hospital they would like to be taken to.
2. Make sure the facility and exercise room are safe and accident free; chairs and steps are not broken, floor is clean, etc.
3. A first aid kit should be accessible to participants and instructors. Instructors and participants should be taught how to use the various items in the first aid kit in case of accident or injury.
4. Have emergency phone numbers of police, hospitals, ambulance, firehouse, administrator and others clearly posted.
5. If a participant does not feel well encourage him/her to sit down and offer a drink of water. While exercising, notice if any participants are being too stressed by the workout. Look for signs such as the face being flushed, profuse sweating from the forehead,

hard breathing, and other symptoms of ill health. See "Fitness —
Minimizing the Risk" page 120 and "Exercise Guidelines"
page 123 for more information on exercise precautions. If a participant gets sick from overworking in the program, the instructor can possibly be held responsible.

6. Always document and report to the facility's supervisor even the
   slightest injury. Each facility usually has its own standard accident documentation form. Keep the accident documentation on
   file for at least one year.
7. Always follow-up on participants who have had an accident in
   the program to see if they have obtained appropriate medical
   treatment.
8. It is recommended that participants have some form of health
   and accident coverage, whether it is Medicare or insurance from
   a private company.

Chapter IV

Program Outline

GENERAL PROGRAM OUTLINE

7:00 a.m. to 8:30 a.m. — set up
8:30 a.m. to 9:00 a.m. — meet and sign in participants
9:00 a.m. to 10:30 a.m. — exercise and health lecture

- exercises (45 minutes): sitting, standing, and brisk walking exercises; exercise routines using broomsticks, frisbees, rubber tubing, light weights
- health lecture/discussion (twenty minutes)
- five minute intermittent breaks

10:30 a.m. to 11:15 a.m. — Participants choice; both sessions conducted at the same time

- active games and sports, or mat exercises possibly concluding the session with a fifteen minute relaxation activity
- swimming and/or water exercises

11:30 a.m. to 12:30 p.m. — optional lunch
11:30 a.m. to 3:00 p.m. — optional field trip every other week to local cultural, recreational, and social centers

The program is normally two and a half hours long (9:00 a.m. to 11:30 a.m.). It can be shortened to two hours without reducing the quality of the program if the instructor is succinct and clear in the activities and exercises.

APPARATUS

For a class of twenty participants, instructor and assistant (twenty-two people exercising):

- forty-four hand-held two pound weights (some preconditioned participants may want to use three pound hand-weights)
- forty-four frisbees
- twenty-two rubber tubing cords
- twenty-two broomsticks
- twenty-two straight-back, nonskid chairs (without arms)
- twenty-two mats, wide and long enough to fully lie down on
- water jug (cooler) and twenty-two cups
- tape recorder with appropriate taped music

STEP BY STEP DESCRIPTION
OF THE "FEELING GREAT!" PROGRAM

Preclass

- Plan out the health lecture or arrange for a guest speaker.
- Photocopy needed information for class.
- Call participants who have missed classes.
- Set up and conduct lectures in the community about the program.
- Do other promotional work as needed.
- Keep an update on monies collected and attendance.
- Go over exercise routines and music to be used in class.
- Attend other exercise classes to learn new routines.

Class, 8:00 a.m. to 8:30 a.m.

- Set out leaflets and resource books in the exercise room.
- Bring out exercise and program equipment such as broomsticks, hand-weights, frisbees, mats, rubber tubing cords, cassette recorder and tapes, water jug and cups.
- set out a circle of chairs in the exercise room and make sure the floor is clean and none of the chairs are broken.

8:30 a.m. to 9:00 a.m.

• Greet new and regular participants coming to class.
• Have new participants complete the registration form and hand out the written materials such as the health evaluation and the exercise booklet, *Pep Up Your Life: A Fitness Book For Seniors*.
• Show participants how to take their pulse and figure out their target heart rate.
• Discuss with volunteer staff and assistant what help you may require today, including the needs and difficulties of some participants.

9:00 a.m. to 10:30 a.m.

Exercise and health lecture: forty-five minutes of exercise, twenty minutes of lecture/discussion, ten minutes of breaks

9:00 a.m. to 9:15 a.m.

• Come into the exercise room, have participants sit in the circle of chairs.
• Introduce new people.
• Tell what the health lecture will be and if any guests will be coming to speak.
• Present announcements concerning participants' health, possible field trips in the near future, and community events.
• Ask if anyone has other announcements or any physical problems or pains requiring some special exercises or attention.
• Review the areas which will be covered in the exercise program:

    1. deep breathing
    2. range of motion, flexibility, stretching
    3. cardiovascular endurance exercises
    4. strengthening endurance exercises
    5. relaxation—visualization, progressive muscle relaxation, deep breathing

• discuss the exercise home program—time, length, and type of exercise. A home exercise program of twenty to thirty minutes twice a day, morning and evening or every other day for 45 minutes is recommended (see page 73 for in-depth home exercise program description).

- review the components of the "Feeling Great!" wellness program:

  1. health care education (see page 74)
  2. proper exercises and relaxation activities
  3. diet/nutrition
  4. peer support/healthy relationships
  5. positive attitude about self, others and life in general
  6. awareness of and responsive to the needs of participants' bodies, minds, and emotions

- have participants take their target heart rate before exercising (see page 112)

9:15 a.m. to 10:30 a.m.

- Begin exercises. A three to five minute standing or sitting *warm-up* to music can be done before introductions to slowly loosen up participants, getting their muscles and body relaxed. *Warm-up* is an essential part of exercising. Gently stretching, bending, loosening up, and possibly lightly jogging in place, slowly warms up the body for more intensive exercising. During the warm-up never bounce up and down because it can cause muscle tears and actually tighten up the muscle.
- Have participants *sitting* in a circle doing *range of motion exercises (head to toe)*, including hand and arm exercises, leg and foot exercises, head and neck stretches, then do body pats "waking up the body."
- Next have participants *stand by their chairs* (with one arm holding onto the chair) and do leg lifts, leg circles, kick backs, short knee bends, and other related exercises. *Do total body stretches*, bends, shakes, shoulder shrugs, *full arm range of motion exercises* (10 times in each direction with each arm).
- Next balance on toes and reach to the sky, and then balance on heels; bend at hips and slowly rotate the hips; and do other stretches and exercises to loosen up the body.
- Everyone takes a *broomstick* and does the stretching and aerobic routine together.

- Next do the *cardiovascular walking routine* — walk fast, change to walking with long strides, change to walking with high steps, change to sliding side to side, change to skipping, change to walking slower, change to walking rapidly, change to walking slowly again (the time length for each segment of the activity depends on the group).
- Next everyone takes a *frisbee* and does the routine together.
- Once the group has exercised enough to get their pulse rates up have them walk slowly and take their pulse to determine their *target heart rate*.
- A *cool down* follows while taking the target heart rate. Have the group walk slowly, breathe deeply, and possibly do some light stretches to enable the body to return to a relaxed state. The cool down helps to circulate the blood back to the vital organs. If participants immediately stop their movement after exercising, the blood which has been vigorously circulating throughout the body will pool in the extremities and can cause physical difficulties such as light headedness, dizziness or fainting.
- *five minute rest*
- *twenty minute health lecture/discussion*
- Rubber tube, walking, and light weight exercises are held next unless the instructor and participants would rather do mat exercises. Mat exercises are very helpful for strengthening the back muscles and for waist, stomach, and thigh exercises.
- Everyone takes a *rubber tube* and does the routine.
- Next do the *walking routine*, followed by exercises with *light weights*.
- *Walk slowly* and *take target heart rates*, then *cool down*. *Cool down* can include slow stretches, relaxing movement, and nonstressful exercises that follow the vigorous exercising.
- *Conclusion of the first part of the group session:*

  - Have group members hold hands and form a circle.
  - Do *stretching* back and forth, side to side.
  - Bend knees slightly and rock back and forth on toes and heels alternately.
  - Rotate shoulders, arms, wrists, and finger joints.
  - Do group activities such as body part to body part game or

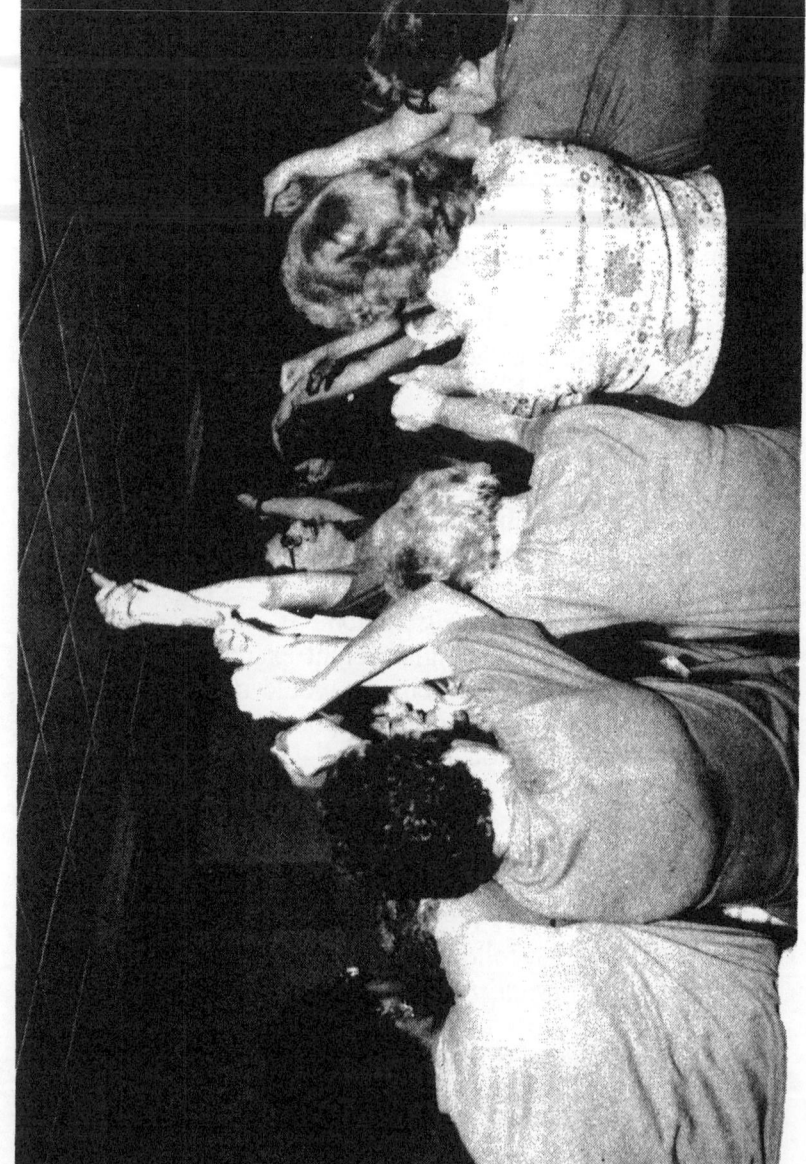

Group cheer at the closing of each class

"massage train." (A "massage train" is when people stand or sit behind each other and massage each others' backs, necks, and arms.)
—With music playing, end with a *group circle activity* such as singing a favorite song or holding hands and coming to the center of the circle with their hands raised saying "yea us" or "Feeling Great!"

Break for five to ten minutes so participants can drink water, socialize, use the bathroom, look over leaflets and books. Those people who will go swimming should now change into their swimsuits. The instructor and participants can set up the mats for floor exercises or prepare for a game activity.

Participants have a choice of either going to the pool to swim or do water exercises, stay in the exercise room for either mat exercises, a game activity, relaxation exercises, or go to the jogging track to do brisk walking.

10:30 a.m. to 11:15 a.m.

Mat exercises and possibly group games: In the last ten to fifteen minutes of the session the instructor may want to conduct a relaxation exercise activity.

10:30 a.m. to 11:30 a.m.

Swimming pool: water exercise, swimming lessons, and free time in the pool

11:30 a.m. to 2:00 p.m.

Optional field trip

EXERCISE HOME PROGRAM

It is recommended that all participants exercise daily or every other day at home to receive the full benefit of the program. All participants are provided with the pamphlet *Pep Up Your Life, A Fitness Book For Seniors*. The instructor can obtain copies of the pamphlet by writing the American Association of Retired Persons, 1909 K Street, N.W., Washington, D.C. 20049. The pamphlet will help participants remember and review exercises they need to practice at home. It is an excellent exercise instruction resource.

Home Exercises

1. deep breathing and relaxation exercises
2. full range of motion/flexibility
3. strengthening
4. cardiovascular endurance

Ideally, full range of motion and flexibility exercises should be done twice a day, once in the morning and once in the evening for fifteen to twenty minutes at a time.

Strengthening exercises and brisk walking or jogging should be done every day or every other day for twenty minutes. These exercises aid in cardiovascular conditioning, endurance, and toning of the body.

For those individuals who claim they do not have enough time to exercise, review a few brief routines which they can do in fifteen minutes. Help them decide on a good time to exercise and how to keep to their exercise schedule.

To make exercising at home more appealing, have participants exercise with a friend or family member. Show participants activities they can do at home which would provide them with a good workout such as exercising with towels, small weights, broomsticks, rubber tubing cords, frisbees, exercising to their favorite music or television exercise show.

The goal participants set out for themselves in the program should directly relate to their exercise homework plan. Monthly review by the instructor of the participants' goals, progress, and updates on their exercise/diet home program is essential.

HEALTH CARE LECTURE SUGGESTIONS

The health care lecture/discussion is an essential and valuable part of the "Feeling Great!" program. The lecture/discussion al-

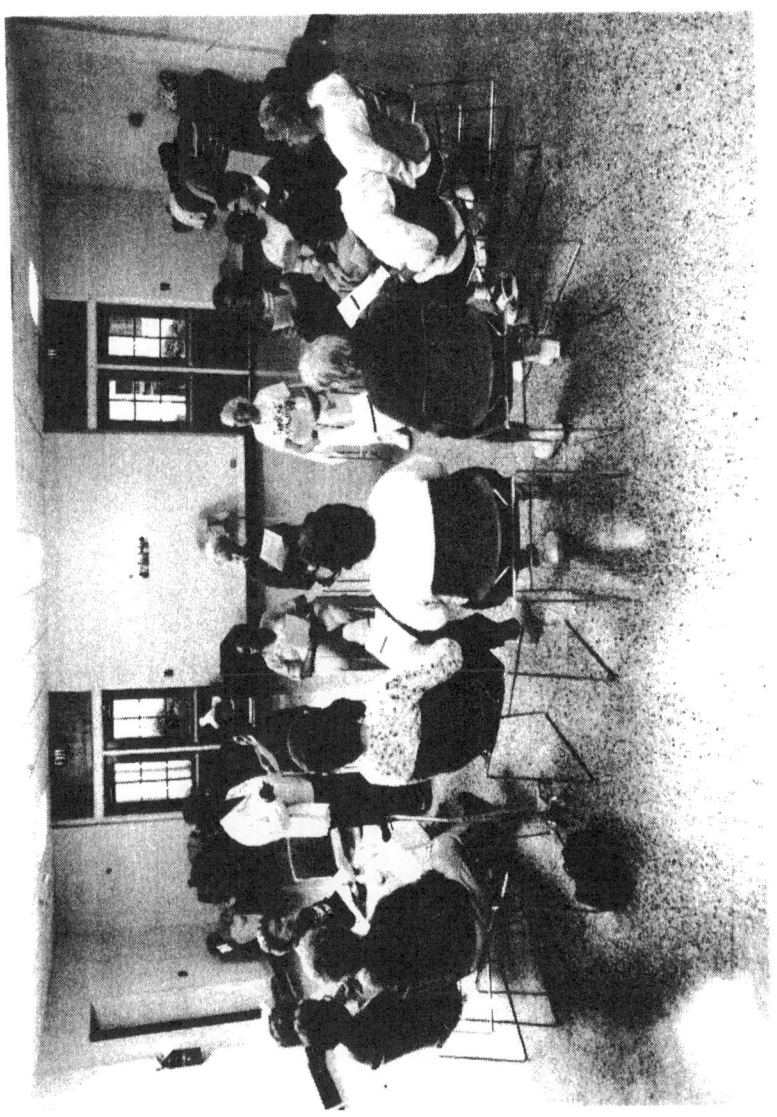

Health care lecture/discussion

lows for participants to learn and share about various physical and psychological health care issues and topics. These discussions can open participants' eyes to new ways of taking care of oneself, inform them of valuable medical check-ups for older adults, good nutrition, and being a wise health care consumer. The health care lecture/discussion is a forum for new ideas: learning, sharing feelings, thoughts, and concerns with their peers. It may be one of the only times some participants will have to focus on learning about different ways to effectively address their health care needs, their emotional needs, and their spiritual needs.

It is recommended that the lectures be no more than 20 minutes long including group discussion, so the lecture will not interfere with the time allocated for exercising. Each health lecture should be accompanied by a handout that is read aloud to the group.

Suggested Topics

General Topics

1. components of a personal wellness program
2. aspects of physical fitness-flexibility, endurance, strength
3. resources in the city for exercise, enjoyment, and learning
4. health risk factors in our environment
5. protecting your home
6. consumer awareness
7. exercise apparel
8. self-defense and crime prevention/awareness

Psycho-Social Topics

1. stress management
2. relaxation exercises (visualization, progressive muscle relaxation, deep breathing)
3. overweight, obesity, and diet
4. dealing with depression
5. motivation
6. loneliness and what you can do for it

7. healthy relationships
8. aging is negotiable
9. individualism and independence
10. healthy attitudes toward life
11. hypochondria
12. support systems
13. retirement—how to make it fulfilling
14. taking care of ill family members
15. crime watch safety

Physical Health Topics

1. arthritis and exercises for relief of pain and joint mobility
2. first aid and CPR
3. pulse rate and target heart rate
4. relieving muscle soreness
5. foot care and proper footwear
6. care and exercises for the back
7. good posture
8. exercising at home
9. effects of exercise on the cardiovascular system
10. exercise precautions in hot weather
11. contraindicative exercises
12. the importance of walking—racewalking for fun
13. dental care
14. diet/nutrition/vitamins
15. the need for calcium
16. the importance of drinking water
17. cholesterol and heart disease
18. medications/use and misuse
19. hearing loss
20. vision loss and other vision problems
21. diabetes
22. controlling high blood pressure
23. massage
24. cancer screening procedures and tests
25. recommended health care screenings for older adults

26. Alzheimer's Disease
27. health care resources, professionals, facilities, and social service agencies

For further references see the section titled "References/Bibliography," page 201.

HEALTH CARE INFORMATION RESOURCES

There are many good exercise and health care articles in newspapers and magazines that are informative and of interest to class members. Participants are encouraged to look for good health care articles and brochures to share with the class. There are also many public and private organizations and companies which offer free health care pamphlets and materials as noted below.

Many of the following resources are cited from the publication *Staying Well, Healthy Activities For Healthy Older Persons* by the AARP, Health Advocacy Services, Program Dept., 1986. These organizations are just a few of the many groups that offer free or low cost health care literature and other materials such as films, slide shows, and posters.

Other suggested resources for health care information are the local chapters of the Arthritis Foundation, Council on Aging, American Cancer Society, American Red Cross, American Diabetes Association, American Heart Association; local hospitals and clinics; local doctors, dentists, pharmacists, nutritionists, physical therapists, exercise physiologists, and other health care professionals; local YMCAs, YWCAs, and Jewish Community Centers; various food companies; and many other community organizations, businesses and professionals.

Suggested Resources

Administration on Aging
330 Independence Ave., S.W.
Washington, DC 20201
(202) 245-0724

(The federal agency responsible for programs under the Older American Act.)

American Academy of
  Ophthalmology
1833 Fillmore Street
P.O. Box 7424
San Francisco, CA 94120

(Provides information on
eye care, cataracts, glau-
coma, etc.)

AARP - American Association
  of Retired Persons
Fulfillment Section or Program
  Scheduling Office or
  Program Resources
  Department or Health
  Advocacy Services
1909 K Street, N.W.
Washington, DC 20049
(202) 728-4450

American Cancer Society
90 Park Avenue
New York, NY 10016
(212) 599-8200

American Council on Alcohol
  Problems
6955 University Avenue
Des Moines, IA 50311

American Council for
  Healthful Living
439 Main Street
Orange, NJ 07050

(offers health promotion
materials)

American Dental Association
211 East Chicago Avenue
Chicago, IL 60611

American Hospital Association
Center for Health Promotion
840 North Lake Shore Drive
Chicago, IL 60611

American Lung Association
1740 Broadway
New York, NY 10019
(212) 315-8700

American Red Cross
National Headquarters
17th and D Streets, N.W.
Washington, DC 20006

American Society for Geriatric
  Dentistry
J. Wendall Lotz, DDS
Ohio State University
305 West 12th Avenue
Columbus, OH 43210

Arthritis Foundation
1314 Spring St., N.W.
Atlanta, GA 30309

Cancer Information
  Clearinghouse
Office of Cancer
  Communications
National Cancer Institute
Bethesda, Maryland 20205
(301) 496-6756

Center for Health Promotion
  and Education
Centers for Disease Control
Center for Environmental
  Health
Atlanta, GA 30333

Dept. of Health and Human
  Resources
Public Health Service
Food and Drug Administration
5600 Fishers Lane
Rockville, MD 20857

Food and Drug Administration
Office for Consumer
  Communications
Room 15B-32 (HFE-88)
Parklawn Building
5600 Fishers Lane
Rockville, MD 20857

Grey Panthers
3635 Chestnut Street
Philadelphia, PA 19104

National Cholesterol
  Education Program
National Heart, Lung, and
  Blood Institute
Bethesda, MD 20205

National Council on the
  Aging, Inc.
600 Maryland Ave., S.W.
Washington, DC 20024
(202) 479-1200

(serves as a coordinating agency of numerous programs and has extensive publications for professionals and consumers)

National Council on Patient
  Information and Education
Suite 1010
1620 I Street, N.W.
Washington, DC 20006

(information on medications)

National Council of Senior
  Citizens
925 15th Street, N.W.
Washington, DC 20005
(203) 347-8800

National Dairy Council
6300 North River Road
Rosemont, IL 60018

(free publications on osteoporosis)

National Health Information
  Clearinghouse
P.O. Box 1133
Washington, DC 20013

National High Blood Pressure
  Information Center
120180 National Institutes of
  Health
Bethesda, MD 20205

National Institute on Mental
  Health
Public Inquiries
5600 Fishers Lane,
  Rm. 15C-05
Rockville, MD 20857

National Mental Health
  Association
1800 North Kent Street
Arlington, VA 22209

National Society to Prevent   (information on eye care)
  Blindness
99 Madison Avenue
New York, NY 10016

Nutrition Information and
  Resource Center
Pennsylvania State University
Benedict House
University Park, PA 16802
(814) 865-6323

Pharmaceutical Manufacturers
  Association
1030 15th Street, N.W.
Washington, DC 20005

President's Council on
  Physical Fitness
  and Sports
400 6th Street, S.W.
Washington, DC 20201

Society for Nutrition
  Education
1736 Franklin Street
Oakland, CA 94612

The American Dietetic
  Association
430 North Michigan Avenue
Chicago, IL 60611

U.S. Department of
  Agriculture
Human Nutrition Information
  Service
Room 360
6505 Belcrest Road
Hyattsville, MD 20782

Villers Foundation
1334 G Street, N.W.
Washington, DC 20005
(202) 628-3030

(provides funding for health care campaigns and other programs to empower older adults)

SAMPLE HEALTH CARE LECTURES

Health lectures on four topics are presented for the readers' interest and use: *Practical Programs To Help Prevent Falls Among Older Adults*, *Home Safety*, *Nutritional Needs Of Older Adults* and *Dealing With Stress*. These lectures are not designed to completely fit in the 20 minutes of time allocated for the health lecture, but rather can be presented over time in a few classes during the health lecture session.

HEALTH LECTURE I

Practical Programs to Help Prevent Falls Among Older Adults

C. Jessie Jones, PhD
Instructor in Dept. of Health and Physical Ed.
University of New Orleans

Falls have long been recognized as a common and particularly hazardous problem for older adults. Falls outnumber all other accidents among the older population. In fact, almost one-third of people over 65 living at home will fall each year. For many older people, the consequence of a fall leaves them with limited functional mobility, dependence on family members for assistance, and possible hospitalization or institutionalization (Tideiksaar, 1986). Fallers are often psychologically affected as well, i.e., lower self-confidence and "postfall syndrome" (a severe tendency to show extreme distress and to clutch and grab when attempting to walk unsupported) (Murphy & Isaacs, 1982; Tideiksaar, 1986). Additionally, falls constitute two-thirds of all accidental deaths among the elderly (Rubenstein & Robbins, 1984). The very grave prognosis of older adults who fall mandates a need for preventive interventions. Indeed, it is easier and financially more beneficial to prevent the complications of falling than to treat them.

Preventability lies first in the identification of variables that predispose elderly persons to falling, and then in the rehabilitation of factors that can be changed. Several studies have shown that predictors highly associated with falls are multifactorial and interactional in nature (Reddy, 1986; Rubenstein & Robbins, 1984; Tinetti, Williams & Mayewski, 1986). There are eight major etiological factors that have been reported to be associated with falls among the elderly; these include environmental hazards, physiological changes due to aging and lifestyle behaviors, neurologic dysfunction, acute and chronic diseases and disabilities (especially cardiovascular and central or peripheral vestibular disorders), drug effects, and psychological and mental status (Rubenstein & Robbins, 1984; Tinetti, Williams & Mayewski, 1986). Some practical programs that could help to prevent falls among the older adults are listed below.

Practical Programs to Help Prevent Falls

Home Safety

Home safety programs can help to identify and correct environmental hazardous conditions in the home. Common home hazards that may cause falls include such things as poor lighting, torn rugs, trailing electrical cords, slippery floors, unstable chairs and tables, cabinets too high and toilets too low.

Safe Use of Medication

The side effects of many drugs have been cited as one of the major causes of falling among older adults (Schwartz & Abernathy, 1987). Adverse effects of some medications can cause drowsiness, dizziness, loss of coordination, impaired vision, orthostatic hypotension making the older adult more vulnerable to falling. Education on the proper use and side effects of such medications as beta blocking agents, diuretics, vasodilators, antidepressants, antihistamines, antipsychotics, anticonvulsants and sedatives could help to reduce falling.

Rehabilitative Exercises

Researchers have found that some factors relative to falling may be remedied through prescriptive exercises by improving stability, coordination, posture and balance (Reddy, 1986; Rubenstein & Robbins, 1984; Tinetti, Williams & Mayewski, 1986). Exercises that strengthen the leg and hip muscles, improve the flexibility of the back, hip and leg flexors and extensors, and activities that are structured to improve posture and balance are encouraged. Listed below are several suggested exercises.

Flexibility Exercises
• foot circles
• foot point/flex
• one-leg bent to chest
• quadricep stretch

Strength Exercises for Legs
(Use with or without ankle weights)
Caution: All strength movements slow in both directions; check posture; avoid upper body bending forward and back; breathe throughout movement; be sure chair is stable and will not slip out. People who have had hip or knee replacements should not perform static one leg balance exercises because it places too much stress on the legs.

- straight leg lifts/forward and back (stand next to the chair)
- straight leg lifts/in and out (stand behind the chair)
- quad leg lifts (stand next to the chair)
- hamstring curls (stand behind the chair)
- tiptoes (stand behind the chair)
- stand up/sit down (very slowly)
- knee lift-ups (sit in the chair)
- one leg lift-up and extend (sit in the chair)

Exercise and Activities to Improve Balance and Posture

Participants need to be instructed and "spotted" through progressive low beam activities. The bean should be approximately 5 inches wide and 10 feet long placed on the floor. Stress "good" posture (use videotaping for participants to view themselves). If participants are afraid of walking on a beam they could begin with a taped line on the floor.
- Walk a beam with arms raised sideward to shoulder.
- Walk to center of beam, slight crouch, turn, and return to starting position.

Place four bean bags two feet apart on the walking board
- Walk the low beam with arms raised sideward to shoulder.
- Walk to center of beam, crouch, turn, and return to starting position.
- Walk forward, step over the bean bags without looking down at your feet, walk on to the end of the board.

Place a bean bag on the top of each hand.
- Walk forward to the end of the board while balancing the bean bags on top of the hands.

Place a bean bag on top of the head.
- Walk the low beam with arms raised sideward to shoulder.
- Walk forward heel to toe to the end of the board.

Place a bean bag on the center of the walking board.
- Walk forward to the bag and crouch down. Do not stoop over! Pick up the bean bag and place it on top of your head. Walk on to the end of the board with the bean bag balanced on top of your head.
- Walk the low beam with arms raised sideward to shoulder.
- Walk backward (slowly) on the beam.
- Walk forward just one-third of the way along the walking board; now turn and walk sideways another third of the way. Turn again and walk backward the rest of the way to the end of the board.
- Walk on tiptoes, keeping center of gravity over the feet.

REFERENCES

Murphy, J. & Isaacs, B. (1982). The post-fall syndrome. *Gerontology*, 28, 265-270.

Reddy, M.P. (1986). A guide to early mobilization of bedridden elderly. *Geriatrics*, 41, 59-70.

Rubenstein, L.Z. & Robbins, A.S. (1984). Falls in the elderly: A clinical perspective. *Geriatrics*, 39, 67-78.

Schwartz, J.B. & Abernathy, D.R. (1987). Cardiac drugs: Adjusting their use in aging patients. *Geriatrics*, 42, 31-40.

Tideiksaar, R. (1986). Preventive Falls: Home hazard checklists to help older patients protect themselves. *Geriatrics*, 41, 26-29.

Tinetti, M.E., Williams, T.F. & Mayewski, R. (1986). Fall risk index for elderly patients based on number of chronic disabilities. *The American Journal of Medicine*, 80, 429-434.

HEALTH LECTURE II
Home Safety

Home hazards account for many injuries and falls to older adults which can be prevented through safety precautions. The booklet, *Home Safety Checklist For Older Consumers*, states, "In 1981, over 622,000 people over the age 65 were treated in hospital emergency rooms for injuries associated with products they live with and use everyday."

The booklets cover areas of the home which should be periodically checked for possible hazards and safety measures. Some of these areas are: electrical and telephone cords; rugs, runners and mats; smoke detectors; electrical outlets and switches; lighting; kitchen area; space heaters; woodburning stoves; and having an emergency exit plan. Practical questions such as "Are the stairs well lighted?" and "Are light switches located at both the top and bottom of inside stairs?" and other recommendations for safety precautions are clearly presented.

The publication *Home Safety Checklist For Older Consumers* was developed by the U.S. Consumer Product Safety Commission in cooperation with the U.S. Administration on Aging. Copies of the booklet can be obtained for free from the U.S. Department of Health and Human Services, Office of Human Development Services, Administration on Aging.

A "Fall Hazard Checklist" distributed by the New Orleans Council On Aging is presented on the following page. This checklist is an excellent form for participants to fill out, discuss, and use as a resource to determine if their home is hazard free.

The booklet, *Home Safety Checklist For Older Consumers* and the "Fall Hazard Checklist" are valuable resources for a health care lecture. Participants can share the information with their friends and relatives and help them make their home safer from possible hazards which can be prevented. Many times, people do not think of home safety until it is too late and an accident has occurred. Be safe! An ounce of prevention can sometimes save a life.

For further safety information, write or call:

U.S. Consumer Product Safety Commission
Washington, D.C. 20207
800-638-CPSC or 800-638-2772

Fall Hazard Checklist

A person's risk of falling is high if any of the following are present:
- History of falls, fainting, or loss of consciousness
- Weakness, dizziness, or balance problems
- Medication therapy for high blood pressure, nervousness, sleep, or depression
- Impaired vision
- Problems with coordination of muscles

Throughout the household, check that the following is in order:

___ 1. Flooring and carpeting are in good condition without protruding obstables that may cause tripping and falling.

___ 2. Lighting is bright and without glare.

___ 3. Nightlights are strategically placed throughout the house, especially on stairways and along routes between bedroom and bathroom. Illuminated light switches are used when possible in similar high-risk locations.

___ 4. Telephones are positioned so that persons do not have to hury to answer a ringing phone.

___ 5. Electric cords are not located in walkways. When possible, they are shortened and tacked down to base boards.

___ 6. Clutter does not obstruct walkways.

Bathroom

___ 7. Railings are installed in the bathtub and toilet areas and are easily accessible for use.

___ 8. A nonslip surface is on the floor of the tub and shower. If a bath mat is used, it is of substantial quality.

___ 9. If a throw rug is used, it has a nonskid rubber backing.

___ 10. Water drainage is appropriate to prevent the development of slippery floors after bathing.

Bedroom

___ 11. Throw rugs do not represent a slip or trip hazard, particulary those en route to the bathroom.

___ 12. Bedside table is present for placement of glasses and other items rather than clutter the floor beside the bed.

Kitchen

___ 13. The floor is made of a nonslip material.

___ 14. Spills are cleaned up quickly to prevent slipping.

___ 15. Cleaning and cooking supplies are stored in locations that are not too high (for shorter persons who would otherwise climb) or too low (for persons who develop lightheadedness after stooping).

___ 16. A high chair is available for doing the dishes.

___ 17. A sturdy step stool is available for reaching high places.

Living Room

___ 18. Throw rugs are not present over a carpet or otherwise scattered about.

___ 19. Furniture is placed in positions that allow for wide walkways.

___ 20. Chairs and sofas are of a height sufficient to permit easy sitting and standing for eldery persons.

Stairways

___ 21. Sturdy railings are provided along both sides of stairways, including the stairway to the basement.

___ 22. Step surfaces are nonskid.

___ 23. Materials are not stored on stair landings or thresholds.

___ 24. When possible, bright nonskid tape is placed at the top and bottom steps to indicate where the steps begin and end.

Outside the House

___ 25. Front and back steps are in good condition. During the winter, sand and/or salt are available for slippery surfaces to ensure safety.

___ 26. Walkways are shoveled free of ice and snow in the winter to prevent slips and falls.

In General

___ 27. Objects should not be carried in such a manner that vision is obscured.

___ 28. Ladders should not be used at all, or if they must be, they are sturdy and positioned carefully, and the top step is avoided.

___ 29. Properly fitting footwear with nonskid rubber soles is worn. "Flats" are preferred to shoes with elevated heels.

HEALTH LECTURE III

Nutritional Needs of Older Adults

Health lectures/discussions on nutrition are an essential part of a wellness program. Nutritional needs and weight loss is a very important and popular subject among older adults. Nutritional information is plentiful and can be found in a variety of resources such as, books, magazines, newspapers, periodicals, government and business consumer information booklets and flyers.

The following sample health lecture is taken from *Jane Brody's Nutrition Book* and the pamphlet *Good Nutrition In Later Years* by Channing L. Bete Co., Inc. I have included discussion items at the end of each lecture segment. The discussion aspect of the health lecture is most important for group sharing and discussing ways to integrate the new learning with their lifestyle.

What Is Good Nutrition? (from the pamphlet Good Nutrition In Later Years)

Good nutrition provides the body with the foods it needs to:
• stay fit
• fight disease and infection
• supply energy for work and play

The body uses the food you eat as a fuel and as raw material for building and maintaining blood, bones and tissue.

Eating right as you get older is up to you!
1. Understand the basics of good nutrition.
2. Plan your diet and budget for healthy eating.
3. Make it a habit to eat right every day.

Balanced diet contains the proper amount of six basic nutrients.
1. *Water* — It is vital for digestion, elimination, and most bodily functions.
2. *Proteins* — They provide amino acids that build and repair body tissue.

3. *Fats* — They supply food energy and essential fatty acids and help carry essential vitamins throughout the body.
4. *Carbohydrates* — Starches and sugars provide energy while cellulose provides bulk to the body.
5. *Minerals* — They help build and maintain bones, teeth, and blood along with being necessary for proper functioning of muscles and nerves.
6. *Vitamins* — They help the body use food properly and regulate the vital functions of the body.

Four Basic Food Groups
The noted nutrients can be found in the four basic food groups. It is important to plan your meals to include these foods in your daily diet.

1. *The meat/protein group* — 2 servings per day to supply proteins, fats, B vitamins, iron and minerals.
One serving equals:

- meat, poultry, fish — 2 to 3 oz.
- dried beans, peas, lentils — 1 to 1-1/2 cups cooked
- peanut butter, nuts — 4 tbsp.
- eggs — 2

2. *The milk group* — 2 servings per day to supply protein, calcium, vitamins A and D, riboflavin and phosphorus.
One serving equals:

- milk — 1 cup
- cottage cheese — 2 cups
- yogurt — 1 cup
- ice cream — 1-1/2 cups (but contains extra calories)

3. *The fruit/vegetable group* — 4 servings per day to supply vitamins A and C, minerals and fiber.
One serving equals:

- leafy vegetables — 1 cup uncooked, 1/2 cup cooked
- green and yellow vegetables, potatoes — 1/2 cup cooked
- citrus and fleshy fruits, berries — 1/2 cup cut up or equivalent

4. *The bread/cereal group* — 4 servings per day to supply protein, vitamins, minerals, fiber and starch.
One serving equals:

- bread — 1 slice, roll or muffin
- cereals — 1 oz. ready-to-eat, 1/2 to 3/4 cup cooked
- pastas — 1/2 to 3/4 cup cooked
- rice — 1/2 to 3/4 cup cooked

Discussion Items:
1. Does your daily diet cover all the necessary nutrients?
2. Activity — Complete a Personal Food Inventory as shown on the following page. List each food consumed in one day including snacks. Then determine the total number of servings of each food group consumed. Finally, noting the recommended servings, determine if there are any additional food group servings needed for a balanced daily diet. The food inventory can also be used to count the daily caloric intake with the help of a calorie chart.

Nutritional Needs Change With Age (from Jane Brody's Nutrition Book, page 408-409)

Calories
The most obvious change occurs in the proportion of the body that's made up of lean tissue — muscle and bone. With age, lean body mass declines and the percentage of body fat increases. Thus, even if you weigh no more at 70 than you did at 20, you're "fatter" at 70. If you maintain a youthful level of exercise as you get older, you can probably slow this trend by keeping your muscles and bones in good shape.

A body having a larger proportion of fat needs fewer calories to maintain itself since fat tissue uses less energy than the same weight of muscle tissue would use. This fact, combined with the tendency of most people to become less active as they grow older, leads to decreased caloric requirement of 2 to 8 percent for each decade of life past 20. This is why many people gain unwanted weight in

PERSONAL FOOD INVENTORY

List below each food consumed in one day including snacks.

Indicate how much of each food you ate such as 2 slices
of bread, 1 chicken leg, 1 cup milk, etc.

Number of Servings

Foods eaten	Meat/ Protein	Milk Group	Fruit/ Veg.	Bread/ Cereal	Other
MORNING:					
AFTERNOON:					
EVENING:					
TOTAL SERVINGS					
MINIMUM RECOMMENDED SERVINGS	2	2	4	4	
ADDITIONAL SERVINGS NEEDED					

middle age. They may eat no more at 50 than they did at 25, but they're less active now and their bodies contain more fat, so they burn fewer calories. If you were maintaining a normal body weight at age 20 on about 2,500 calories a day, by the time you reach 50, you may need only 1,950 to 2,300 to maintain the same weight.

But although you need fewer calories, your need for vital nutrients doesn't diminish significantly. Therefore, you have to pack the same amount of nutrients into fewer and fewer calories as you get older. This means there's less room in your diet for foods that are overly refined, calorically dense, and nutritionally deficient – that is, junk foods. As you grow older it's critically important to make all your calories count, nutritionally speaking. Too often, however, exactly the opposite occurs. As elderly people develop problems chewing and digesting their food, they lean more and more heavily on soft foods of uniform texture – usually food high in sugar and/or fats and low in proteins, vitamins, minerals, and fiber.

It's not a good idea, on the other hand, to overeat just to consume the required nutrients. Keeping your weight down as you age is especially important because extra pounds cause unnecessary stress on your bones, adding to the risk of fractures. Also, obesity contributes to the development of diabetes, heart disease, and high blood pressure, and is an indirect cause of accidents.

Discussion Items:
1. Have participants share their experiences of how easy it is to gain weight and hard it is to lose weight.
2. Talk about the problems and reasons for overeating or eating poorly such as boredom, depression, loneliness and stress. Discuss the problems of consuming too much junk food at home and at fast food restaurants, and the problems of eating and cooking alone.
3. Discuss diet/nutritional plans and where to buy good fresh fruits, vegetables, meats, and seafood that are reasonably priced.
4. It can be lonely for people to eat alone especially if they are divorced or widowed. Discuss the possibility of participants inviting a friend from the program to join them for a meal at a restaurant or to invite someone from the group to their home for

a meal. If participants begin to invite friends to their home for a meal or if they go out to eat, the instructor may want to inform the group of the friendly gatherings to encourage more socialization. At times, the whole class may want to go somewhere for lunch after the exercise session, or go to dinner and a movie together.

5. Discuss places to eat out where senior citizens can get a discount. Also, give class members information on nutrition programs such as: senior citizen congregate meal sites in the community; supplemental commodity programs; the requirements to obtain food stamps and where to register for them; and "Meals on Wheels" which brings food to homebound senior citizens.

6. Discuss food/nutrition problems:

   a. Difficulty chewing foods—A problem for people who have poorly fitted dentures or other oral problems. If it is a problem with dentures, first try to have them corrected. If this does not solve the problem then try eating baby foods. Select those of "pure" ingredients—jars of meat, vegetables, and unsweetened fruits. They will provide balanced nutrients if they are consumed in adequate amounts.

   b. Digestion—With age, the body becomes less efficient at digesting food. Constipation, heartburn and bloating may occur. You can prevent these discomforts by eating smaller meals, more frequently; drinking plenty of fluids; eating more fiber (whole-grain breads and cereals, fruits and vegetables); and eating more slowly and chewing food thoroughly.

   c. Weight control—There are many different recipes for weight control. Some basic suggestions to follow are:

      • Cut down or cut out high calorie foods such as candy, pastries, junk food, and alcoholic beverages. If you do not have them in your home you will not be tempted to eat them as often.

      • Keep a variety of nutritious, low-calorie foods at home such as fruits, vegetables, fish, poultry, low-fat milk, low-fat cottage cheese and low-fat yogurt.

      • Drinking 6 to 8 glasses of water a day can help with weight loss. Drinking cold water is preferred because it is absorbed into the system more quickly than warm water. The body will not function properly without enough water and cannot metabolize stored fat efficiently. Retained water shows up as excess weight but in order to get rid of excess water you must drink more water (Robertson, D., 1986).

- Do not go on a diet but fix the one you have got. The problem with most diets is that they may require drastic changes in eating habits which a person may do for a short time but in the long run it may be too unsatisfying for the individual to practice faithfully. To lose weight on a permanent basis it may be wiser to slowly change eating patterns and food choices. Be informed and aware of the nutritional value and the caloric amount of what you are eating. Make a list of food priorities, plan meal menus and stick to them by keeping a daily log of what you have eaten and the caloric amounts. Discuss your diet progress and difficulties with a friend. This should be a person who can motivate and support you especially when you feel frustrated or upset. It may be better to discuss this matter with only one or possibly two friends so the diet does not become a soap opera but rather a discipline of wise and healthy living.
- People do not plan to fail, they just fail to plan.

d. Iron supply — Insufficient iron in a person's diet can lead to anemia, leaving a person feeling weak, tired, and less able to care for him/herself. It is important to have iron rich foods in the diet such as lean red meat, liver, leafy green vegetables, enriched whole-grain breads and cereals, dried fruits, and legumes.

e. Calcium — Inactivity coupled with a lack of calcium and vitamin D in the diet may lead to weakened, brittle bones and an increased risk of fracture. Osteoporosis is an age-related bone disorder characterized by progressive weakening of the bones. This disorder cannot be cured but it can be treated through exercise, calcium/vitamin B supplements, and diet. A person's diet can help this problem by avoiding the "bone robbers" such as caffeine and large quantities of protein, alcohol, or carbonated beverages and including more foods in their diet which contain calcium such as nonfat dry milk, plain low-fat yogurt, sardines, swiss cheese and cooked broccoli.

HEALTH LECTURE IV
Dealing with Stress

Stress is an anxious feeling that touches everyone sometime in their lives. When the brain perceives a stressful situation, it stimulates the nerves and hormones which cause the muscles to tense, the heart rate to increase, and the blood pressure to rise. If the body is continually under stress without relief, it can make a person feel tired and drained, while creating high blood pressure.

Stress affects people in different ways. Some people thrive on it and are motivated by the stressful challenge that stimulates them to grow and develop and others are devastated by it. When a person cannot cope due to a stressful situation he/she can either try to avoid the stressful situation or learn how to cope.

***Early Warning Signs of Stress (from the book
Is It Worth Dying For? by Dr. Robert
S. Elliot and Dennis L. Breo, pages 19-21)***

Are you under too much stress? Are your friends and coworkers? Air Force psychologist Capt. Neil S. Hibler has developed a list of early warning signs:

Emotional signs
• Apathy — the "blahs," feelings of sadness, recreation is no longer pleasurable.
• Anxiety — feelings of restlessness, agitation, insecurity, sense of worthlessness.
• Irritability — feeling hypersensitive, defensive, arrogant or argumentative, rebellious or angry.
• Mental Fatigue — feeling preoccupied, having difficulty concentrating, trouble in thinking flexibility.
• Overcompensation or denial — grandiosity (exaggerating the importance of your activities to yourself and others), working too

hard, denying that you have problems, ignoring symptoms, feeling suspicious.

Behavioral signs
- Avoiding things—keeping to yourself, avoiding work, having trouble accepting responsibility, neglecting responsibility.
- Doing things to extremes—alcoholism, gambling, spending sprees, sexual promiscuity.
- Administrative problems—being late to work, poor appearance, poor personal hygiene, being accident-prone.
- Legal problems—indebtedness, shoplifting, traffic tickets, inability to control violent impulses.

Physical signs
- Excessive worrying about or denial of illness
- Frequent illness
- Physical exhaustion
- Reliance on self-medication, including overuse of drugstore remedies like aspirin
- Ailments—headache, insomnia, appetite changes, weight gain or loss, indigestion, nausea, nervous diarrhea, constipation, sexual problems.
- Sleeping excessively

No set number of these symptoms indicates difficulty in coping with stress. If you have a combination of these warning signs and have had them over a long period of time, you should talk with a counselor or your doctor about what is bothering you.

Managing Stress

Each person experiences some stressful situation each day. Stress is not a negative word. In fact, stress can be defined as a challenge in life. Too little challenge leaves a person bored and stagnant; too much creates a feeling of overload and out of control. A healthy amount of challenge spurs a person on to develop talents and gain a sense of accomplishment and purpose.

The individual's perception of a stressful situation and how he/she deals with it is the major factor of how it will affect the person's life. A major question to ask concerning coping and stress is: Are individuals controlled and burdened by their stress or do they have some control over the level of stress and know how to handle the stress?

Managing stress is managing the anger and anxiety people feel in stressful situations so that they can work toward solving the problem creatively. It is regaining a sense of balance and control in the situation by either changing conditions in the environment or changing expectations or perceptions of the situation.

Creative problem solving means being flexible yet resilient, with the ability to view the situation, develop options and follow through with a new strategy. For example, two people can be in a similar stressful situation. In dealing with the situation one person may become physically upset and ill, while the other person, having better coping skills, is not overwhelmed and can rise to the situation in order to seek a solution. Some tips on how to prevent stress overload:

1. *Listen to your body*. When you feel tired, do not keep pushing — rest. When you feel tense, find a way to relax.
2. *Prepare for change*. In today's society there is nothing more certain than change. So expect it and be ready for it. Your expectations or hopes may not be fulfilled. Anticipate the opportunities and problems that might come along in your daily life along with knowing what resources and support systems you have.
3. *Manage your time*. Define your priorities. Plan how you will use your time each day. List what you want to accomplish. Decide what is more important and do those things first. Do not let others tell you how to spend your time. Learn to say no.
4. *Learn to get along with others*. Build a support system with friends, family, and coworkers. Develop a team spirit in your life by sharing ideas and involving others in your plans.
5. *Put balance into your life*. Avoid becoming isolated or a workaholic. Make time for yourself, family, friends and activities.
6. *When facing a stressful situation, ask yourself the following questions:*

    a. Can I change something in my environment to make the situation less stressful?

   b. Can I adapt or change my way of handling the situation to make it more tolerable?

   c. Can I avoid the situation, and for how long?

   d. What is the worst and best that can be expected out of the situation and how will that effect me?

   e. What are my needs in the situation and what are my options, resources, supports, and abilities in handling the situation?

   f. If I could change the situation in any way possible how would it change and what are the needed steps to make the change a reality?

7. *Exercise* helps to lower blood pressure and may reduce the "stress chemicals" currently present in the body (Eliot, R., 1984). Stretching and aerobic exercise can also release tensions in the body due to stress. Exercise may relieve some feelings of depression and anxiety, and can increase an individual's sense of self-control and self-esteem.

   Exercise helps your heart and lungs work better. As your heart, lungs and circulatory system improve, a number of good things happen. Nutrients and oxygen move more easily to all parts of your body. Wastes are removed more efficiently. Your enzyme system stays in better balance, so your muscles can relax more completely. You sleep better, and your endurance increases (Tubesing, 1981). The benefits of exercise culminate in an increased sense of well-being.

8. *Massage* aids in relaxing tension and helps a person to feel physically better which can then help the individual to look at his/her situation in a new light.

9. *Spiritual consolation* through a person's faith and support from fellow members of his/her religion can often motivate and offer a new perspective, and shed a new "light" on the situation. The religious beliefs and practices of older adults are often a very important part of their lives.

Discussion Items:

1. Have participants discuss the stressful situations they encounter and how they deal with them, such as dealing with grief, loneliness, moving, losing a friend, money problems, problems with friends and/or family.

2. Discuss different ways of coping. How to use inner resources and social supports. Recommended book for instructor and participants, *Is It Worth Dying For?* by Dr. Robert S. Eliot and Dennis L. Breo.
3. Discuss the importance of exercise in reducing stress.
4. *Activity* — Have participants role play a stressful situation dealing with a family member. After the role play have participants discuss the different ways to handle the situation.
5. *Activity* — Have participants role play a stressful situation dealing with money. After the role play have participants discuss different ways to handle the situation.

Stress is a fact of life.
Manage it,
Don't let it manage you.

Chapter V

Exercise Outline

PHYSICAL FITNESS

According to the President's Council on Physical Fitness and Sports (*The Fitness Challenge in the Later Years*, June 1984), physical fitness is the ability to carry out daily tasks with vigor and alertness, without undue fatigue and with ample energy to engage in leisure time pursuits and to meet the above average physical stress encountered in emergency situations.

Components of Physical Fitness

1. *Flexibility*: ability to move a joint through a full range of motion.
2. *Muscular strength*: the capacity of a muscle or muscle group to exert a force against a resistance.
3. *Muscular endurance*: capacity of the muscle to exert a force repeatedly over a period of time or to hold a fixed or static position for a period of time. It is the ability to use strength and sustain it over time.
4. *Cardiovascular endurance*: a measurement of the body's ability to take in, transport, and utilize adequate amounts of oxygen to the working muscle, allowing activities that involve large muscle masses (such as walking, jogging, bicycling, and swimming) to be performed over long periods of time.
5. *Relaxation*: the ability of the body to release muscular tension as well as change other physiological and cognitive stress responses.

FIVE IMPORTANT PHASES OF EXERCISE ROUTINES

1. *Warm-up phase*: A warm-up period consists of low-level exercise activity moving each part of the body through the full range of motion. It provides the body with a gradual adjustment in the circulatory system and a gradual increase in muscle and body temperature which prepares muscles for more vigorous activity.

2. *Muscular strength and endurance phase*: There are two types of muscular strength and endurance activities — isometric and isotonic exercises.

   Isotonic exercise is a dynamic contraction in which the muscle is allowed to shorten such as in rubber tubing and light weight exercises, weight training and calisthenics.

   Isometric exercise is a press or a pull against immovable objects. People who have high blood pressure are advised not to use this type of exercise activity because it can easily elevate their blood pressure. For this reason the "Feeling Great!" program does not use isometric exercises.

3. *Aerobic phase*: Aerobic activity involves the use of large muscle groups, continuously exercising in a rhythmic manner for a sustained period of time. Examples of aerobic activities are jogging, walking, biking, and swimming. These activities utilize oxygen in the production of energy for muscular contraction. The aerobic activity elevates the heart rate into the training range (60-80% of age adjusted heart rate).

4. *Cool-down*: This is a gradual recovery from the workout using walking, and other low-intensity exercises. These activities permit the gradual circulatory readjustments, and allow the dissipation of body heat. They prevent the pooling of the blood in the extremities and the rapid fall in blood pressure after vigorous exercise which can trigger dizziness and possible fainting.

5. *Static Stretching*: After exercising the muscles are warm and primed for proper stretching activities to allow for maximum flexibility and range of motion. Stretching helps to maintain joint mobility and flexibility.

DEVELOPING A PERSONAL FITNESS PLAN

The following material is adapted from the *YMCA Corporate Health Enhancement Program*, edited by William D. Zuti and Cole Mandelblit, 1980, National Board Of Young Men's Christian Associations.

It is important that participants receive proper guidance and support at the beginning of joining the exercise program. Exercise guidelines (see page 123) and fitness recommendations as noted below should be discussed.

1. Most people can undertake an easy moderate exercise program without risk. But, caution is advised before advancing to a more vigorous exercise activity. It is recommended to have a medical examination before beginning a rigorous cardiovascular or muscular endurance program.

2. Some people enjoy group activities but should not limit their exercises to these activities alone. It is most important to take time daily for some structured exercise activity and to integrate more activity into their daily routine. Some suggestions include:

    a. Whenever possible use the stairs instead of taking elevators or escalators.

    b. If they have a habit of sitting a lot or perform an activity in which they must sit for a long period of time, make sure to take periodic breaks to stand, breathe deeply, stretch, and walk around. Consider standing during phone conversations and doing abdominal or stretching exercises.

    c. After breakfast or lunch make it a routine to take a brisk walk.

    d. Sometimes it is enjoyable to make a change in the exercise activity because variety makes the activity more interesting. If participants enjoy the exercise activity they will make an effort to be consistent in their practice and consistency is a key to success.

3. Remind participants to start off slowly and to increase gradually within their own limits. Most people have spent years getting

out of shape. They should not presume that they can get back into shape in a few days. Have participants begin at a safe and comfortable intensity and duration of exercising and then gradually progress as their body develops its level of conditioning.

4. Remind participants whenever exercising to always begin exercise activity with a warm-up and end with a cool-down and stretch for proper exercise precautions.

5. Most authorities feel that 40 minutes to an hour of exercise every day is highly desirable. But, participants must do what is comfortable for them, even if it is only five to twenty minutes of exercising. It may be helpful to break up the exercise routine by warming-up for five minutes, vigorously exercising for five to fifteen minutes, then cooling down for five minutes, followed by vigorous exercise for five to fifteen minutes, then cool down for another five minutes.

6. Participants should be advised about proper eating habits such as controlling the consumption of fats, sugars, and calories as needed. Also eating before exercising should be limited and drinking of water before and after exercising encouraged.

7. Have participants be realistic and optimistic in their expectations. Remind them that many of the changes they will experience from exercising are physiological and not externally visible right away. Judge the success of the program and their participation on how good they feel and not just how much weight they lost or muscle they gained.

8. Remind participants it is essential to maintain a consistent exercise program rather than a sporadic attempt to get in shape which often proves unsuccessful.

9. Participants should determine personal objectives, goals, a time frame, and a personal action plan to meet their fitness goals (see Contract/Goals Form and Goals, Homework, Periodic Review Form pages 181 and 180).

10. If after exercising individuals feel excessively tired during the day they should cut back on their exercise activity to a comfortable level and try to slowly build up their strength and endurance. If they continue to be tired throughout the day from their exercise activity they should then consult their doctor. Exercise should make a person feel more alert and invigorated. For those

people who are very out of shape exercise can tire them until they build up their stamina and strength.

11. Proper footwear for all exercise is essential for support, to prevent injury and for good posture.

STRETCHING

The following material is adapted from the book *Stretching* by B. Anderson, Shelter Publications, 1980. This publication is an excellent resource for instructors and participants.

There are two types of stretching, ballistic and static stretching. *Ballistic stretching* involves quick, jerky, bouncy movements which can damage muscular-skeletal tissue and is not recommended for exercising. *Static stretching* is steady, relaxed, and sustained stretching with limited movement.

There is a right way and a wrong way to stretch. The right way is a relaxed, sustained stretch with your attention focused on the muscles being stretched. The wrong way is by bouncing or lengthening and shortening the muscle abruptly during exercise. Also, stretching to the point of pain can be harmful and is not recommended.

There are two phases of proper stretching, the easy stretch and the developmental stretch. The *easy stretch* is a slow deliberate lengthening of the muscle or muscles to the point where resistance is met and tension starts to build. This stretch should be held from 10 to 30 seconds without bouncing. Have participants stretch to the point where they feel a mild tension and then relax as they hold the stretch. The feeling of tension should subside as they hold the position. The easy stretch reduces muscular tightness and readies the tissues for the developmental stretch.

After the easy stretch move gently into the *developmental stretch*. Once a muscle has adjusted to the first phase, the easy stretch, then the second phase or developmental stretch lengthens the muscles slightly, but not to the point of great pain. Stretch slightly until the person feels a mild tension again and hold for 10 to 30 seconds. During this time the tension should diminish or ease off slightly. The developmental stretch fine-tunes the muscles and increases flexibility.

It is essential that participants breathe slowly and rhythmically while stretching and do not hold their breath. With feelings of slight tension or pain, *breathing* can help reduce the pain by refocusing on the breathing pattern. Also, counting the seconds while stretching will ensure that participants hold the proper tension for the needed length of time and help to refocus them away from the mild tension or pain.

The muscles are protected by a mechanism called the *stretch reflex*. When the muscle fibers are stretched too far either by bouncing or overstretching, a nerve reflex responds by sending a signal to the muscles to contract, which keeps the muscles from being injured. Therefore, when people stretch too far they tighten the very muscle they are trying to stretch. This is why it is important to have a sense of balance, control, and awareness of the body to know how much to stretch and when to relax.

Benefits of Stretching

Proper stretching will help individuals to increase their range of motion through smooth articulation of their joints. Stretch before and after each workout to loosen and relax the muscles. Stretching reduces muscle tension and helps the body feel more relaxed. It helps in coordination by allowing for freer and easier movement, good posture and balance, and aids in developing body awareness. Stretching promotes good circulation and feels good!

Stretching Guidelines

1. We may feel different every day. Some days we are more tight or loose than other days. Have participants notice and be aware of how their bodies feel on various days. Also, notice the difference the weather can make in the way a person feels. On a rainy day participants may feel stiffer from the dampness in the air and they may have more arthritis pain. On a sunny day they may feel lighter and more relaxed.
2. Do not stretch too far in the beginning, but remind participants to gradually increase their stretch as they progress in their conditioning.

3. Try not to have participants compare themselves with each other. Proper stretching means stretching within their own limits, relaxed, and without comparisons. Even if they are tight or inflexible, do not let that discourage them from stretching and improving. Try to notice the day-to-day small positive changes that occur from the stretching exercises.
4. Have participants breathe slowly, deeply, and naturally as they stretch. Remind them not to stretch to a point where they cannot breathe easily.
5. Participants should focus on the areas of their body which they are stretching. If the tension becomes greater as they are stretching, they may be overstretching and should ease into a more comfortable position.
6. Regularity in stretching along with relaxation of the muscles after stretching are essential factors in a healthy workout.
7. Be very cautious when stretching muscles that surround painful joints.

CARDIOVASCULAR FITNESS AND TARGET HEART RATE

Beginning a safe, individualized and progressive cardiovascular exercise program can be accomplished by following three fundamental steps:

1. Begin by having a thorough medical examination which should include a stress test. A stress test may use a treadmill, stationary exercise bicycle, or the doctor may instruct the patient to walk over some steps or jog in place to measure the performance of the heart while it is exerting itself, such as during exercise. This test can measure heart rate, blood pressure, oxygen use, and monitor the electrical impulses of the heart by taking an electrocardiogram (Cooper, 1985). For some individuals cardiovascular exercise might not be safe. It is possible to feel good and have no major outward signs or symptoms and still suffer from coronary-artery disease. Cardiovascular exercise or strenuous activity could aggravate a pre-existing condition and possibly cause serious problems.

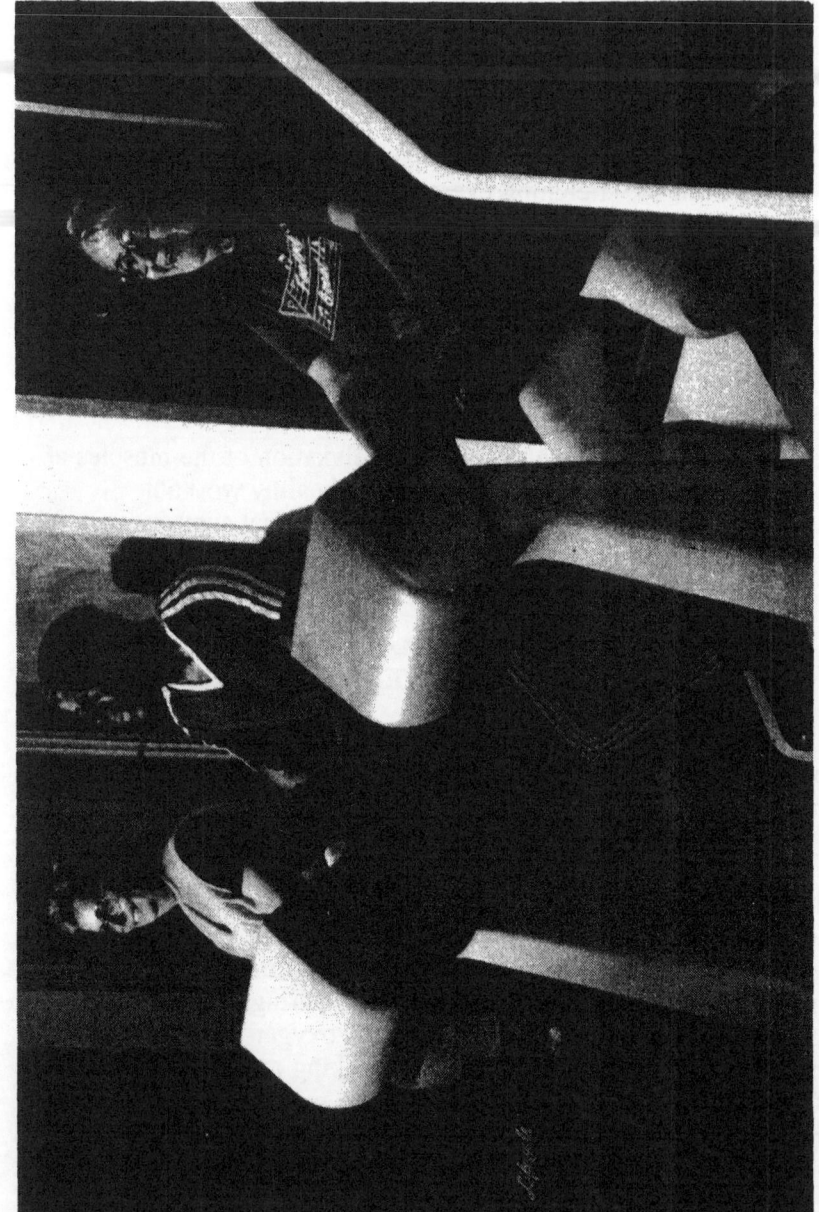

Cardiovascular exercise on exercise bicycles

2. Participants should know their target heart rate and monitor it while exercising. Because the heart rate is related to the intensity of the exercise as well as the oxygen consumption, by monitoring the heart rate participants will know whether their pace is too fast or slow for proper exercise conditioning activity. It is generally agreed among fitness experts that to get an appreciable training effect from exercise, the heart rate should be between 60% and 80% of the predicated maximum heart rate for the individual based on his/her age. This range is known as the target heart rate zone. The training target heart rate for beginners should be between 60% and 70%, with gradual increases as they develop in their cardiovascular fitness conditioning. Some preconditioned participants may exercise as high as 85%, though this is not necessary for training effect.

a. Finding the target heart rate (training rate):
  • Participants should learn how to take their pulse (heart beats per minute) either on the wrist with the middle two fingers or on the carotid artery in the neck while walking during the cool-down portion of the exercise activity. Once participants can determine their pulse they can then find the target heart rate. It is very important to slowly cool down after exercising and not stop or sit down immediately after the activity to insure the bodies' slow readjustment.
  • To find the maximum heart rate, participants should subtract their age from 220 beats per minute. To find the target heart rate multiply this number by 60% and 80% which provides the lower and upper ranges of intensity for their aerobic exercise.

Example: for a person who is 60 years old—

220	160	160
− 60 years	× .60	× .80
160	96.00	128.00

The range is 96 to 128 heart beats per minute or 16 to 21.5 heart beats per 10 seconds.
b. Checking the training or target heart rate—Immediately after exercising have everyone take their pulse for 10 seconds. Multiply this number by 6 to calculate how many times their heart

Target Heart Rate Chart

10 Second Count

Age	60%	80%
40	18	24
45	17.5	23.5
50	17	22.5
55	16.5	22
60	16	21.5
65	15.5	20.5
70	15	20
75	14.5	19.5
80	14	18.5
85	13.5	18

Participants need to consult their physician before beginning a cardiovascular exercise program. Senior Citizens should not increase their heart rate to the target heart rate zone before prior progressive aerobic training and conditioning with the guidance of a certified exercise instructor.

The Exercise Activity Pattern

Resting	—	Warm-Up	—	Vigorous Activity	—	Cool Down	—	Relaxation
		5 - 10 Minutes Pulse Rises		20 Minutes Enter Target Heart Rate Zone		5 - 10 Minutes Pulse Lowers		

has been beating per minute during exercise. Use either the pulse in the wrist or the carotid artery in their neck.

3. Choosing the right cardiovascular activities is very important. The mode of exercise outside of the "Feeling Great!" class should be safe but at the same time challenging enough to the cardiovascular system. It should be a convenient accessible activity that participants can enjoy spending approximately two hours per week doing (a minimum of a thirty minute session every other day). The more convenient, accessible, and fun the activity is, the more the individual will want to continue to exercise regularly. If the activity takes a lot of preparation, or participants have to go a long distance to get to the activity, they may become more easily discouraged from frequent exercising. Participants should carefully plan how they can incorporate their leisure exercise activities into their daily life.

Some examples of the most popular activities which improve cardiovascular fitness are: brisk walking, jogging, swimming, cycling, aerobic dancing, and roller skating.

When starting the cardiovascular program, participants should keep the intensity and amount of time spent at their chosen activity low (5 to 15 minutes at 60 to 65% of maximum heart rate). Have participants progress to a more intense level only after they have gradually conditioned themselves over a period of time.

A safe way to introduce cardiovascular fitness exercises into a program with people who are "out of shape" is to begin by exercising at slow speeds for 5 to 15 minutes and then taking a short break. After participants have been able to build their exercise intensity to a comfortable level, slowly increase the length of time exercising. While doing cardiovascular-aerobic exercises, participants should be able to talk with no strain. If they are not able to talk comfortably while performing light aerobic exercises, they may be pushing themselves too hard.

Some warning signs of when to stop cardiovascular exercising are when a participant breaks out in a cold sweat, becomes faint, or has chest pains. If participants are taking high blood pressure medication they should exercise slowly so they will not dramatically increase their blood pressure which their medication is trying to control. A well structured exercise program three times a week can help to lower an individual's blood pressure. The main idea in exercising is to progress slowly, toning up the body and strengthening the cardiovascular system.

EXERCISE POINTERS FROM THE YMCA PROGRAM
"TWINGES IN THE HINGES"
AN EXERCISE PROGRAM FOR PEOPLE
WITH ARTHRITIS

Use It or Lose It
Exercises for Your Arthritis

Often, one of the most important things participants can do to help their arthritis is to exercise.[1] Unfortunately, many people with arthritis think exercise is harmful. Others become discouraged because progress is slow. Maintaining a proper balance between rest and exercise is the key to a successful arthritis exercise program. Examine the following benefits of exercise, some basic principles, and the different types of exercise.

Benefits of Exercise

There are numerous physical and psychological benefits of exercise. It is well-known that exercise leads to increased strength and flexibility in the muscles and ligaments surrounding the joints. In addition, research has shown that exercise, such as swimming or walking, has important effects on the heart that promote increased endurance and circulation and fights deterioration of the arteries.

Every tissue in the body requires certain foods or nutrients to work effectively. Most tissues have arteries that bring essential foods to them, but this is not true of the joint cartilage. It is only through movement that nourishment is brought by the synovial fluid to the joint cartilage thereby removing the waste products. Thus, exercise promotes good joint nutrition. An exercise program can lead to a general sense of well-being and accomplishment. It is easy

---

1. Includes material from the brochure *Twinges In The Hinges, An Arthritis Aquatic Program Especially For People With Arthritis*. Co-sponsored by the Memphis YMCA and the Arthritis Foundation.

for people to feel good about themselves when they are accomplishing the goals of a realistic exercise program.

Furthermore, the social interactions encouraged by the program are also rewarding in themselves. Exercise is a way we can prevent the loss of function that may accompany arthritis. There is a saying that applies particularly to persons with arthritis: "Use it or lose it." If you do not use a muscle or joint you will lose strength and mobility, and thus function. If loss of function has already occurred, it is important to remember that it was not lost in one day. Likewise, it cannot be regained in one day. Slow progress is to be expected, particularly if the arthritis is severe or the joint limitations have existed for a long time. But, most often, any efforts will be well rewarded in many ways.

Principles of Exercise

When Should Participants Exercise?

Exercises should be done daily for the rest of your life. It is the "weekend warrior" who gets in trouble with painful strained muscles and ligaments. It is better to exercise at a slow, steady rhythm, giving your muscles time to relax between each repetition. Make sure you do not bounce when exercising because that will only tighten the muscles and can possibly tear the muscle. The only time a joint should not be exercised is when it is inflamed, or "hot" (swollen, red, or tender to the touch). The "hot" joint is one of the special exercise considerations for people with rheumatoid arthritis. However, even these hot joints should be gently moved through the full range of motion twice a day. In osteoarthritis, there is a noninflammatory slow degenerative effect upon the joint cartilage, accompanied by bone and cartilage thickening or overgrowth. Though there is minimal inflammation involved with osteoarthritis, there often is a lot of pain in the joints that limits the range of motion; the hands are the most afflicted area (C. J. Jones, 1986). With osteoarthritis, exercise is essential to decrease stiffness and to prevent loss of range of motion.

Participants should make exercise a part of their daily routine. They will have to decide on the best time, but consider the following: It is best to exercise when (1) they have the least pain, (2) they have the least stiffness, (3) they are not tired, and (4) their medication is having maximal effect.

How Should Participants Exercise?

Be consistent and attend the chosen exercise classes regularly along with exercising once or twice daily at home to maintain joint mobility. Have participants begin at a level which is comfortable for them and then gradually increase the number of repetitions. Explain that they should progress slowly when having rheumatoid joints that are prone to "hot" periods. With this gradual progression, they will avoid unnecessary pain. Heavy and resistant activities should be avoided with people who have arthritis. Rather flexibility exercises and mild dynamic stretching movements that include all parts of the body with good posture can be extremely effective in reducing pain and improving joint mobility. Have participants coordinate their breathing with the exercises. By counting the exercises out loud together it can help participants breathe deeply and regularly. One way to psychologically help participants who suffer from arthritis pain is to practice breathing out the pain and breathing in the healing, while exercising.

The instructor should know about participants' limitations, disabilities, and when participants are suffering from arthritis or other physical problems. This will enable the instructor to aid participants in performing selected exercises.

Types of Exercise

There are three basic types of exercises.

Range-of-motion or stretching exercises involve moving a joint as far as it will comfortably go and then coaxing it a little farther, just past the point of beginning pain or discomfort. These exercises are designed to increase and then maintain joint mobility, thus decreasing pain and improving function.

In normal activities of daily living such as housework, bathing, cooking, and walking, people usually do not use a full range of motion of the joints which is focused on in exercise classes. Therefore, daily activities will not give the individual the complete exercise benefit an exercise program can offer.

Strengthening exercises increase muscle strength and thus lend stability to vulnerable joints. They improve participants' ability to bear weight, lift objects, and sustain movement. Strengthening exercises should be done in such a way as to minimize stress on the joints. Remember, strengthening exercises are not a substitute for stretching exercises. They will not increase joint range of motion.

Endurance exercises are necessary because neither stretching nor strengthening will increase endurance. More dynamic forms of exercise, such as walking, swimming, bicycling, jogging, dancing, or cross country skiing will promote cardiovascular fitness. Participants should include some kind of dynamic exercise in their program every day, but they should remember to start out easy and progress slowly. To help reduce stress while walking or dancing, wear low-heeled, rubber-soled, light weight shoes. A good running shoe is essential for any runner with joint or muscle problems; try them on before you buy and consult a running guide for current recommendations. These are often excellent shoes for just walking.

FEAR OF EXERCISE: EXERCISE FOR THOSE PEOPLE WHO ARE OUT OF SHAPE AND FOR THOSE WHO HAVE SOME PHYSICAL PAIN

Fear of exercise for older adults occurs for various reasons. These reasons can arise from physical difficulties and/or emotional apprehensions. It is important for the instructor to be aware of older adults' fears towards exercising. It is very helpful if the instructor designs individualized "home-practice" programs which deal specifically with the participant's needs, along with motivating the individual with a positive attitude toward exercise. The instructor must keep in mind any physical risk which may confront participants while exercising.

In many cases when certain body movements cause people pain they often restrict their activities which can eventually undermine their ability to regain greater functioning, instead of developing their bodies to its highest level of functioning. If people who have some physical difficulties restrict their activities to a very sedentary level they can lose much of their muscle tone, flexibility, and their joints may stiffen up.

Physical Aspects of Exercise for Those with Special Problems

Older adults who have gone through a major operation such as a hip replacement may find themselves with limited mobility and a fear of exercising and even possibly injuring themselves. It is imperative that these individuals speak to their doctor about their need to exercise to increase and develop their physical abilities and ask what special precautions they should follow or be aware of while exercising. The doctor may also be able to recommend particular exercises to do or avoid.

Often when people begin an exercise program they experience some muscle discomfort, especially those who have pain from arthritis or people who have not exercised in many years. This is normal due to the strain on unexercised muscles.

When exercising and experiencing pain it is advisable to go slow or even temporarily stop the particular activity until enough strength and flexibility is developed to begin the exercise without major discomfort. Slight discomfort from one exercise should not prevent an individual from performing other exercises. The exception is when they have symptoms of a heart attack such as chest pain, heart pain, or a pain radiating down the left arm. Anyone having these symptoms should stop exercising immediately and consult his/her physician.

It is important to design a personal exercise and nutrition program, with the help of a licensed exercise instructor and nutritionist, to meet the individual's needs. For those adults who are disabled, recovering from illness or injury, or for those people with chronic problems it is necessary to consult one's doctor on recommended exercises and those exercises to avoid. Even people who are wheelchair-bound can still stretch and exercise most muscles without getting out of their chairs.

Exercise needs to be a part of the individual's everyday life, like eating food. While it is beneficial and motivating to exercise with a group, it is also essential for participants to continue to exercise daily. Exercises such as brisk walking, chair exercises, and flexibility can easily be done everyday within participants' daily activities. The excuse of not having enough time to exercise should not come up, if participants' daily activities are arranged to incorporate various sitting, standing, and walking exercises. The extra time put in daily exercising will make participants physically more comfortable and possibly more satisfied in their life.

Emotional Aspects of Exercise for Those with Special Problems

It may be true that it is hard to be motivated to exercise when a person is out of shape or is not accustomed to exercising, and especially if he/she has some pain with physical movement. It is also usually certain that a sixty-year-old person who is overweight and out of shape will probably not be able to exercise and diet to such an extent as to look like the magazine models who are in their twenties and thirties. But what is the consequence of not taking good care of the body through exercising and eating properly? Many people suffer from not exercising and the cost is poor health. The adventure and enjoyment of getting into better shape, breathing better, having more energy, feeling more flexible, alive, and welcoming every new day is the beauty of being involved in a personal fitness program.

Fitness, for participants who are disabled or have some physical pain means making strides to develop their cardiovascular conditioning, flexibility, and strength throughout the whole body from head to toe regardless of the possible limitations. Though participants may become discouraged at times and have some setbacks, remember nobody's perfect and no body's perfect!

A good attitude is crucial to the success of an exercise program. A positive attitude toward exercising and an understanding of the components of wellness enable participants to strive to be the best they can be. A positive attitude can replace the discomfort, discouragement, and difficulty of exercise with hope for the future. Have participants create a vision of how they want to feel and look after exercising and as they progress they may possibly even go beyond their personal conception of wellness.

When participants have a vision they can strive for, temporary setbacks can more easily be accepted while creatively looking for new ways to get in shape. As the old expression goes, where there is a will there is a way. We must aspire to be the best we can be. In this process participants may find that they can become even greater, grow healthier, improve their physical condition and increase their awareness and joy of life. The benefits of their efforts can be experienced in all aspects of their lives, such as, new relationships, interests, and an increased sense of self-esteem. The more participants work toward their goal, the deeper their commitment, while the benefits from their efforts multiply.

It is impossible to anticipate how much better participants will feel from the benefits of the program because they may have never taken the opportunity to exercise on a regular basis. Due to changes in their lives, senior citizens may now have more free time to exercise, regulate their diet, and try things they did not have a chance to do when they were working a full-time job. Paradoxical as it may sound, participants usually have more energy after exercising than they did before the activity. Like any piece of fine machinery, the body works better when it is used regularly and taken care of. By exercising participants will have more strength, flexibility, and energy to fill their day. This will enable them to enjoy more enriching activities in their lives.

FITNESS—MINIMIZING THE RISK

Awareness

Have participants be attentive to the signals (feelings) in their body. Participants should notice their breathing. Are they breathing hard? Participants should be able to talk comfortably while doing aerobic exercises. Are participants sweating, and is it throughout the whole body or only on their head? People who have high blood pressure may break out in a cold sweat on their forehead if they exert themselves too much. Do participants' complexions change color to red or white? If it does they may be working out too hard. Do they feel any pains in their chest, stomach, or other parts of their body? Do they feel dizzy, lightheaded, or nauseated as they exercise? These symptoms are warning signals to either slow down or stop exercising. Class members need to be aware of their bodies' needs and be able to adjust their exercise routine to suit their abilities and limitations.

What Are the Signs of Injury or Overexertion?

Stiffness in a joint, tingling, numbness or swelling, or pounding in the heart, extreme breathlessness, nausea, chest pain, or trembling are among the warning signs that a participant has forced his/her body past conditioned limits. When participants feel these symptoms or a pull, twist or strain, have them *stop exercising immediately* and rest till the pain subsides. Continuing to exercise can make the injury worse. If the pain subsides and they start exercising again upon which the pain worsens, have participants stop exercising.

If an injury occurs, participants can minimize the damage with the well-known formula, RICE, which stands for rest, ice, compression, and elevation.

Rest: It is most important to rest following any type of injury. If the injured part is not rested and is subject to external stress and strain, the healing process can be impaired.

Ice: For sprains, much of the pain and swelling can be prevented by the immediate application of ice packs, which will constrict some of the smaller blood vessels and reduce internal bleeding (Memmler & Rada, 1970). Wrap ice in a towel or place in a plastic bag, or use an ice pack or a bag of small frozen vegetables and place on the injured area for 20 to 30 minutes.

Compression: Compression helps in controlling swelling. Compression helps to reduce the amount of swelling by applying pressure around the injured area. Pressure can be applied by using an elastic wrap (such as an Ace bandage) with firm but even pressure around the injured area (Prentice & Bucher, 1988).

Elevation: The injured area, particularly an extremity, should be elevated to eliminate the effects of gravity on blood pooling in the extremities.

For relieving painful joints various methods can be used such as: a heating pad; a hot-water bottle; a towel soaked in hot water, wrung out and placed on the affected area; and even a hot bath (Frank & Frank, 1972). When using a heating pad, keep it at a low heat setting and apply it to the joint for 15 to 20 minutes.

For further information on first aid refer to the American National Red Cross, *Standard First Aid And Personal Safety* manual.

When Is It Time for a Doctor?

The instructor should provide participants with some guidelines as to when it is necessary to see a doctor for physical problems. With any new injury or significant physical pain that does not subside, participants should notify their physician. Some other reasonable guidelines are:

- An injured part does not heal itself or function properly.
- The neck, head, or back has received a strong blow.
- A head injury is accompanied by dizziness, impaired vision and/or severe headache.
- Chest pain, shortness of breath for an extended period of time, arrhythmias (irregular heart beat)
- Feeling nauseous whenever moving
- Other related problems

COMMON PHYSICAL PROBLEMS
AND INTERVENTIONS WHEN EXERCISING

Major chronic physical problems should be diagnosed by a physician who will advise what exercises should be done and what exercises are to be avoided. If any exercises cause pain, the participant should immediately stop doing the particular exercise and notify the instructor. If pain is severe or recurrent, the participant should consult with his/her doctor.

1. *Problem* — lower back pain
   Intervention — When exercising bend knees, keep the legs parallel and the back straight. Many of the mat exercises are excellent for strengthening the back. Refer participants to also join a YMCA's "Y's Way to a Healthy Back" course.

2. *Problem* — knee pain
   Intervention — Do full range of motion exercises three times a day, slowly exercising the joints. Walking and practicing mat exercises builds up knee strength. Do not perform a lot of bouncing activities as it puts extra weight on the joint momentarily without strengthening the legs. Some knee problems can get worse from exercise and participants with knee problems should consult with their doctor before starting an exercise program.

3. *Problem* — limited ability to walk
   Intervention — Do some of the exercises in chairs, others holding onto a chair. Practice walking till you are too tired or have pain. Daily, practice balancing, flexibility, and agility exercises. Three times a day do full range of motion exercises. Mat exercises can help strengthen the legs.

4. *Problem* — limited range of motion of joints
   Intervention — Three times a day do full range of motion exercises from head to toe sitting in a chair and then standing next to a chair; possibly holding onto the chair when needing extra assistance in stability.

5. *Problem* — unable to get onto a mat on the floor without assistance
   Intervention — Learn the correct way to bend down, to get onto the floor, and to stand up. Practice balancing and agility exercises and other exercises which will strengthen the ankles and legs.

6. *Problem* — assorted physical problems including arthritis
   Intervention — Water exercises are good for many physical problems because the buoyancy of the water takes the weight off weight-bearing joints making them easier to move and exercise.

EXERCISE GUIDELINES

In older adults the joints, tendons, and ligaments move less freely and are less elastic. Their bones become more brittle and can break more easily and their muscles lose some of their strength. But, with proper exercise all of these losses due to aging can be minimized (Grey, 1985).

In order to best help the participant, an instructor needs to be a careful watcher, a good listener, and an excellent teacher. Instructors must make sure the participants are learning and performing the exercises correctly, not overdoing the workout, or lacking in their participation. Noted below are a few guidelines to assist instructors in the intricate process of leading an exercise program with older adults.

General Instructor Guidelines

1. Help participants to try new activities or those they felt they could not do. Help them to overcome fears they may have of physical activities through support, guidance and learning how to exercise properly. Be patient and allow time for participants to possibly work through any fears of physical fitness. Encourage exercising at a moderate pace on a regular basis and slowly work through any fears of exercising.
2. As you perform the exercises, inform participants how their bodies are benefiting from the activity. Explain why each exercise is done and the differences they should feel during and after exercising. Keep these talks short and to the point. When participants can see the immediate benefits of exercising, they will be more motivated to continue.
3. It may be helpful to some participants to aid them in adjusting their diet to include more nutritious foods or delete unnecessary sugars and fats. Point out how the effects of exercise, diet, and a healthy attitude about themselves can change their lives in a positive direction.
4. Point out to participants that excess weight will create extra strain on their joints which can increase their arthritis pain and possibly reduce their flexibility.
5. Use the expertise of other fitness professionals in the community to assist you in making your class the finest. You are providing a tremendous service to your participants. Make sure the class is the best it can be!
6. Some participants may have trouble hearing or seeing, so in-

YMCA OF GREATER NEW ORLEANS

CONTRAINDICATIVE EXERCISES *

To prevent muscle soreness—or even worse effects—the YMCA feels that certain exercises should not be performed by the average person.

Avoid at all costs any bouncing and jerking exercises that force the joints to the limits of their range of motion. Indeed, you should never do any exercise at any time that puts unnatural pressures on body parts. For instance, doing exercises that put a pulling pressure on the spine and neck or place lateral pressure on a joint that does not naturally move in that direction is asking for trouble. There are plenty of other exercises available to give you the most complete workout possible without running the risk of injury.

There are seven exercises in particular to be avoided by the average person. They are: (1) the Yoga Plow, which puts unnatural pressure on the neck and back; (2) the Hurdler's Stretch, for which the knees must bend unnaturally; (3) the Duck Walk and Deep Knee Bend, which puts too much pressure on the knees; (4) the Stiff-Legged Toe Touch, a traditional exercise that puts great strain on the knees and back; (5) Ballet Stretches, which should be only for trained dancers because it puts too much strain on the ligaments, knees and lower back; (6) the Stiff-Legged Double Leg Raise, which is an old-line calisthenic that puts too much strain on the lower back; (7) the Stiff-Legged Full Sit-Up, which strains the lower back.

Double Quad Stretch No-No

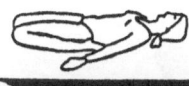

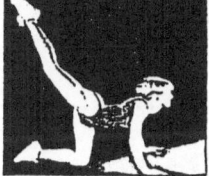

Donkey Kicks No-No

• Avoid hyperextending the cervical and lumbar spine.

• Do exercises and stretches in a way that won't cause stress on the joint. There is usually an alternative way to do the same exercise or stretch.

• Work on muscle balance of antagonist (opposite) muscle groups. Example: Everyone does lots of work on abdominals, but they lack low back strengthening. This causes muscle imbalance which can lead to injury.

• Use proper alignment of the exercise to get the specific muscle you are aiming for.

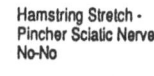
Hamstring Stretch - Pincher Sciatic Nerve No-No

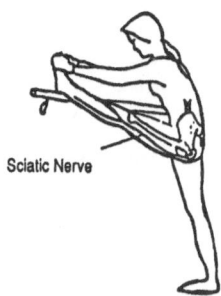
Sciatic Nerve

---

* From The Official YMCA Fitness Program by William B. Zuti, Ph.D., Rawson Associates, New York, 1984. Pages 37-39, including additional material by the YMCA of Greater New Orleans.

A "No - No" Exercise
Yoga Plow — It puts
unusual pressure
on the neck.

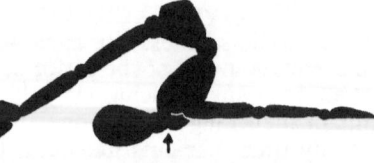

A "No - No" Exercise
Hurdler's Stretch — It
puts unnatural pressure
on the side of the knee.

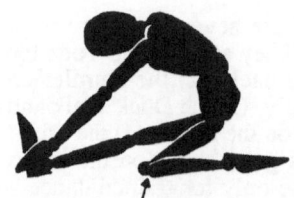

A "No - No" Exercise
Duck Walk and Deep Knee
Bend — It puts too much
pressure on the knees.

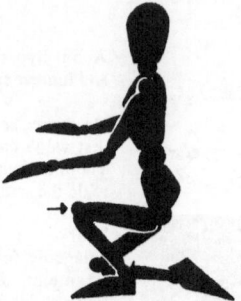

A "No - No" Exercise
Stiff Legged Toe Touch —
It puts too much strain on
the back and knees.

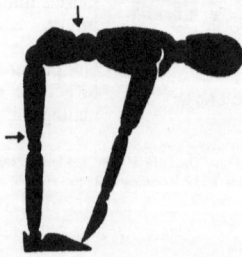

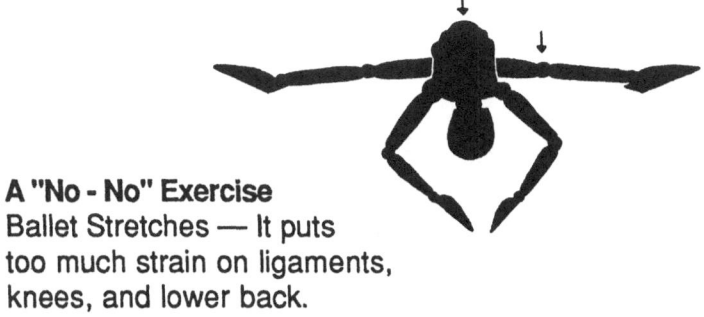

A "No - No" Exercise
Ballet Stretches — It puts
too much strain on ligaments,
knees, and lower back.

A "No - No" Exercise
Stiff Legged Double Leg
Raise — It puts too much
strain on the lower back.

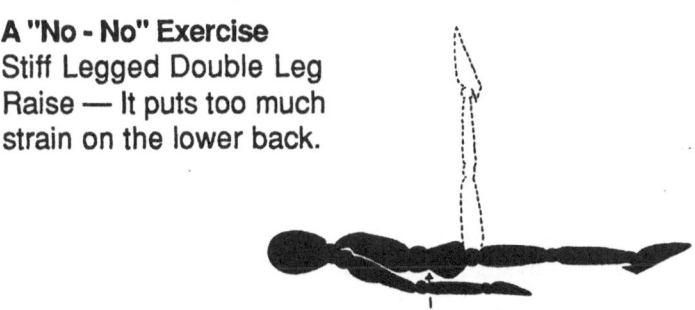

A "No - No" Exercise
Stiff Legged Full Sit Up —
It puts too much strain on
the lower back.

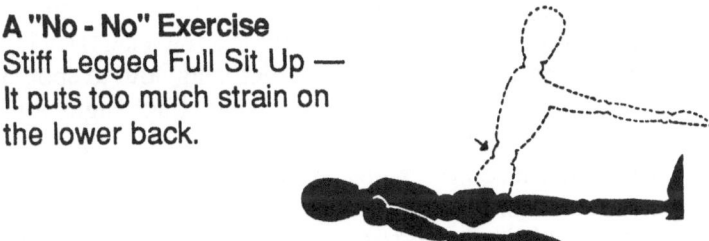

Also avoid hands behind the head pulling on the head,
which stresses the cervical spine.

structors should always position themselves so they can be easily heard and seen by the group. Watch for facial and postural signs that point to participants who feel left-out, very tired, in pain, or who want to exercise more.

7. For some participants who are out of shape it may be necessary to physically help them by assisting in moving their limbs through the full range of motion until they learn to do the exercise by themselves properly.

Guidelines Specific to the Exercise Activity

1. Encourage participants to have the proper dress for exercising which consists of shorts or jogging pants, tee-shirt, sweatshirt, and a good pair of aerobic or walking exercise shoes. A good shoe is essential and most important to prevent injuries and to give the foot proper support. For some people a high-top shoe may be more comfortable because of the support it lends to the ankles. A good shoe (sneaker) should have a stiff heel cup and a cushioned inner sole made of durable, spongy material that absorbs the impact of jumping.

2. Know the physical limitations of class members and obtain an intuitive sense of how much participants can exert themselves. Watch for body and facial signals from participants to see how much they can do comfortably. Allow people to slow up whenever they want to, to speed up or do more repetitions of an exercise if desired. Do not perform too few exercises in fear of overworking the class. Teach participants how to spot signs of when to slow down or stop exercising. Such signs are: being out of breath, having chest or stomach pains, having strong leg pains, experiencing cramps, or any unusual pain. Always ask participants for feedback concerning whether the exercises are too fast, too slow, too strenuous, not strenuous enough or just right. Never be a mind reader, have the participants tell you how they feel.

3. At first keep the number of repetitions small (five), but once participants have practiced for a while increase the number of repetitions. Allow those who are in better shape to do more exercises.

4. Exercise at a slow, steady rhythm, allowing participants' muscles to relax between each repetition. It is best to exercise at a comfortable pace with good posture, going through a full range of motion, developing endurance rather than speed. Consistent patterned exercises are fun when done to music, making the exercise pattern fluid and easy to follow.

5. If a participant is afraid of falling, especially if he/she had fallen before, let the person do many of the exercises sitting, standing by the chair, or by a rail to hold onto if his/her balance becomes shaky.

6. Jogging is ill advised for people who have knee, foot, or related joint problems. These individuals can obtain the cardiovascular benefit of jogging through brisk walking.

7. Coordinate breathing with the exercise and remind participants not to hold their breath when exercising. If participants cannot carry on a conversation or are gasping for breath while they are doing aerobic exercises, they are probably exercising too hard.

8. Teach participants the correct way to do certain activities without straining the body such as to bend down, to reach for something, to briskly walk, and other common physical movements. Remind participants when exercising to keep their knees slightly bent and their backs straight so they will not strain their backs when stretching or reaching. Before performing any floor exercises, instruct participants on the correct way to sit down and get up from the mat.

9. Begin each class with a three- to five-minute warm-up, gently swinging arms, stretching the arms, legs, and back, rotating the hips, bending with the knees flexed, and other related exercises. This activity enables the muscles to warm and the joints to rotate to prepare the body for more vigorous exercises.

10. Cool down — After the vigorous phase of exercising, slowly do stretching and moving exercises for three to five minutes. After the peak portion of exercising, make sure participants do not stand still, do not sit, nor stand motionless while taking their pulse. Make sure they keep on walking, stretching and moving during the cool-down while checking their pulse. Make sure they do not start talking and forget to keep on moving to *slowly* bring the body back to rest. The cool down is an essential as-

pect of the exercise process. Exercising without cooling down is similar to driving a car and coming to a dead stop, which can be very harmful to the body.

11. Check target heart rate twice in each class.
12. Encourage those participants who exercise on a regular basis to try to gradually increase their workout.
13. Try to make sure participants enjoy the exercises and activities. If they do not enjoy the activities they probably will not do them at home on a regular basis.
14. Show how participants can feel some improvement in each class. Make sure the exercises are not too difficult for participants to succeed in the program.
15. Remind participants that they may be younger than someone else in class but not able to exercise at the same intensity due to individual limitations and conditioning. Each participant needs to exercise at his/her own level and intensity. The class is a supportive environment not a competitive one.
16. Muscle strain frequently involves the back muscles. To avoid muscle strain of the back muscles remind participants that while exercising to keep their back straight, their knees slightly bent, and to not perform any fast action jerking movements.

Guidelines for the Class Setting

1. The exercise room should be well lit and air conditioned/heated. It should be a pleasant room with a clean floor and should have a clock with a second hand so participants can check their target heart rate whenever needed. It is best to exercise on wooden or hard rubber floors, or plastic-covered foam mats because they cushion the impact, to some degree, of the participants' movement as opposed to cement or tile floors which are totally resistant to pressure. Consistent aerobic exercising on cement or tile floors can hurt participants' feet or knees.
2. A first aid kit should be readily accessible to the instructor and participants. Also, a list of emergency phone numbers such as the police, fire department, ambulance, hospitals, and facility administrator should be posted.

3. Chairs — Make sure the chairs have straight backs, no arms, and nonskid feet.

- Teach participants how to sit erect in chairs — good posture is very important. Also, instruct members on the correct way of bending down to sit and get up.
- Begin the class with sitting exercises — range of motion, flexibility, hands, feet, and facial exercises.
- Use the chairs for support and safety in exercising.
- Chairs are especially helpful in bracing oneself when standing up. Have chairs nearby for rest periods. If participants can only stand for a limited amount of time due to knee, leg, or joint problems allow them to do some of the exercises sitting in chairs and some while standing and holding onto the chairs.

4. Regular participation should be encouraged and home exercising on a daily basis stressed for maximum benefit. Program benefit will come best from consistent practice.

5. Allow opportunities for social interaction before and after class. During class, it is advisable to sometimes have participants teach a few exercises or have them show each other the correct way to do some exercises. Discussion among participants about health problems and ways to deal with those problems should be encouraged as a group learning, sharing, and peer support activity.

6. Always select music according to the tempo of the exercise. Using a range of music styles from rock, to country, to classical music makes the class more interesting, varied and meets the interests of more people. The instructor may want to use contemporary music which he/she enjoys. If the instructor is motivated by the music then he/she may find it easier to motivate participants.

7. The group is comprised of people with different abilities. Have those individuals who are in better shape encourage and assist those who are not in as good physical condition. Let participants provide motivation for each other in the class. *We are not just growing older, we are growing better!*

8. For participants who have handicaps, modify or alter the exercises for their needs and abilities. Be creative in discovering

ways in which people can exercise. Do not single out the handicapped person in an embarrassing manner.

9. Each person is at a different level of physical ability which can either hamper or help the group activity. The more physically fit members can assist others while still being committed to their level of exercise intensity. This can build the spirit of camaraderie and fellowship in the program. It is important for Seniors to be role models for each other. In the group activity, the instructor should make it seem like everyone is working together at the same level though in reality everyone is exercising at a little different pace to meet their own needs.

10. When asking class members how they enjoyed the program be aware that they might not tell the truth because they may feel it would hurt the instructor's feelings. The participants may be very sensitive to not wanting to reject the instructor or feel rejected themselves.

FITNESS LEADERSHIP

Individuals interested in leading exercise programs should be trained and certified by a local YMCA in "Fitness Leadership." The exercises listed for the "Feeling Great!" program can be fully described and taught in a YMCA instructor training session.

For a list of training workshops contact the "YMCA Active Older Adult Program" at 1-800-USA-YMCA. To receive a newsletter on YMCA older adult programs, the "YMCA Active Older Adult Program Memo," write to Mary Howell, Editor, AOA Program Memo, YMCA of the USA — Program Services Division, 101 North Wacker Drive, Chicago, IL 60606.

Exercise Instructor's Role

It is important for instructors to be aware of their communication with participants and their verbal and nonverbal response. Some senior citizens may have limited contact with others and a limited amount of things to do during the day so these individuals may spend many hours or days thinking about what the instructor had said in the class. In this regard, instructors need to be aware of what they say, how they say it, and the participants' response.

Instructors have a great responsibility to the health and well-being of their class. Being "up," inspirational, friendly, touching, holding hands, patting people on their backs and saying a few kind words to each participant aids in recognizing their involvement in the program and is one key in reaching the hearts of the participants.

If the instructor is tired, not exercising regularly, not eating well, or mentally preoccupied, his/her class can suffer. Participants will consciously or unconsciously pick up the notion that the instructor has low energy or interest in the program and they may choose to socialize more and possibly be less attentive to the exercises. Though any instructor at times can become tired or overworked which can interfere with the session, the instructor can tell the class of his/her feelings and either ask one of the participants to lead the group, or request the group to continue exercising to their full capacity while the instructor may slow down.

It is imperative that the instructor also be committed to a personal exercise program, watch his/her diet, and try to put his/her full energy into the program. The instructor is the role model, motivator, and facilitator of the program. His/her enthusiasm can lift the spirits of participants who may be unsure of themselves in the program. The instructor is one of the keys to the program, helping participants to learn about exercising, dieting, eating correctly, feeling, and thinking about the world in a new way.

HANDLING DIVERSE ABILITIES
AND INTERESTS IN A GROUP

For most participants the class's primary goals vacillate between an exercise/health education program and an opportunity to have a very pleasant social time. Both goals are vital ingredients of the program, but it is important to make sure one goal does not totally outweigh the other.

The program is designed to allow participants to work up to their full capacities. For some people that may be just seven exercise repetitions and for others it is fifteen exercise repetitions. To enable a group of people with diverse abilities and disabilities to exercise together, everyone begins each exercise activity together but counts out the repetitions to themselves (striving to do ten repetitions). This allows each person to go at his/her own pace and enables participants not to feel pressured to do the same amount of exercise as others. Sometimes it is helpful to count the exercise repetitions out loud to build the group spirit and to try to have everyone working together.

If exercise repetitions are not counted aloud, some group members may primarily focus on the social aspects of the group and may not exercise to the degree needed to provide an optimal workout. On the other hand, too much emphasis on keeping up with other class members can make the program too inflexible and demanding. A careful balance needs to be achieved.

It is important and basic to the program to stress the use of good posture, moving gracefully, using their full body correctly in all types of exercise and movement. Good posture helps in having a positive self-image which is one of the valuable goals of the program.

MUSIC

Music played throughout the exercise session can help participants by giving them a beat to exercise by and providing enjoyable background sounds. Varied styles of music from rock and roll to ethnic or regional music to classical music can be used as long as it fits in with the exercise and the participants enjoy the sound. Using the same music can help participants in their exercise routine because they have grown accustomed to the beat and are familiar with the sound.

Contemporary music can work well with a senior citizen group if it is introduced enthusiastically and suits the exercise pattern. From my personal experience of using rock and roll music because it is personally invigorating, I have found that many participants who originally disliked the music, over time, learned to love it. In fact they would not exercise without the usual rock and roll music playing. Some participants even bought cassette tapes of the rock and roll music to exercise with at home because it reminds them of the group and the exercise activity.

APPARATUS AND ACTIVITIES
USED WITH BASIC EXERCISE PATTERNS

As the instructor develops knowledge of flexibility, endurance, and strengthening exercises he/she will be able to design exercise routines using the various apparatus described below.

1. *Type of exercise* — flexibility, range of motion
   Examples — static stretching, exercising through the full range of motion, water exercises
   Apparatus — broomsticks, frisbees, swimming pool
2. *Type of exercise* — coordination/reflex exercises/balance/agility
   Examples — ball games, patterned exercise movements with and without apparatus
   Apparatus — broomsticks, frisbees, ball games, various movement patterns
3. *Type of exercise* — cardiovascular endurance exercises
   Examples — brisk walking-jogging, swimming/water exercises
   Apparatus — safe place to walk/run, swimming pool
4. *Type of exercise* — muscular strength and endurance exercises
   Examples — lifting light weights and pulling rubber tubing as resistance for strengthening key muscles
   Apparatus — light one, two or three pound weights, rubber tubing

FITNESS EXERCISES

Within the following pages, the "Feeling Great!" exercise routines are briefly summarized. The exercises noted are only a basic overview of some of the movements of the exercise routine to familiarize the reader with the program. The book, *The Official YMCA Fitness Program* by William B. Zuti, PhD (1984), depicts and explains many of the exercises cited. But, it is best to learn exercise leadership from a certified instructor.

Many older adults joining an exercise program may not have exercised in many years, their bones are more fragile and often they are not as flexible as in their youth. Therefore, it is most important to caution participants to do the exercises correctly to prevent any possible injury. The author does not recommend for the reader to merely look over the exercises and begin teaching them to older adults without a proper course and certification in fitness.

Exercises Described:

1. Chair exercises
2. Standing exercises
3. Walking exercises
4. Frisbee exercises
5. Broomstick exercises
6. Rubber tubing exercises
7. Hand-weight exercises
8. Mat exercises
9. Swimming and water exercises
10. Active games
11. Relaxation exercises

Reminder: Whenever an exercise is done with one side of the body, repeat the exercise on the other side to get a full workout and to prevent building up only one section of the body. Remind participants who have a strong dominant side, such as being either right or left handed or having a stronger leg, to also exercise and build up the weaker side.

CHAIR EXERCISES

Teach participants the proper way to sit in chairs to exercise with their back straight, feet and legs parallel, both feet on the floor, and arms at their sides.

Activities: five to ten repetitions depending on the individual; perform repetitions slow and deliberately.

• Begin by taking three deep breaths, slowly breathe in and expand your chest and then slowly breathe out, continue to inhale and exhale with each exercise.
• Hold arms by the side and do arm circles, first in one direction and then in the other direction.

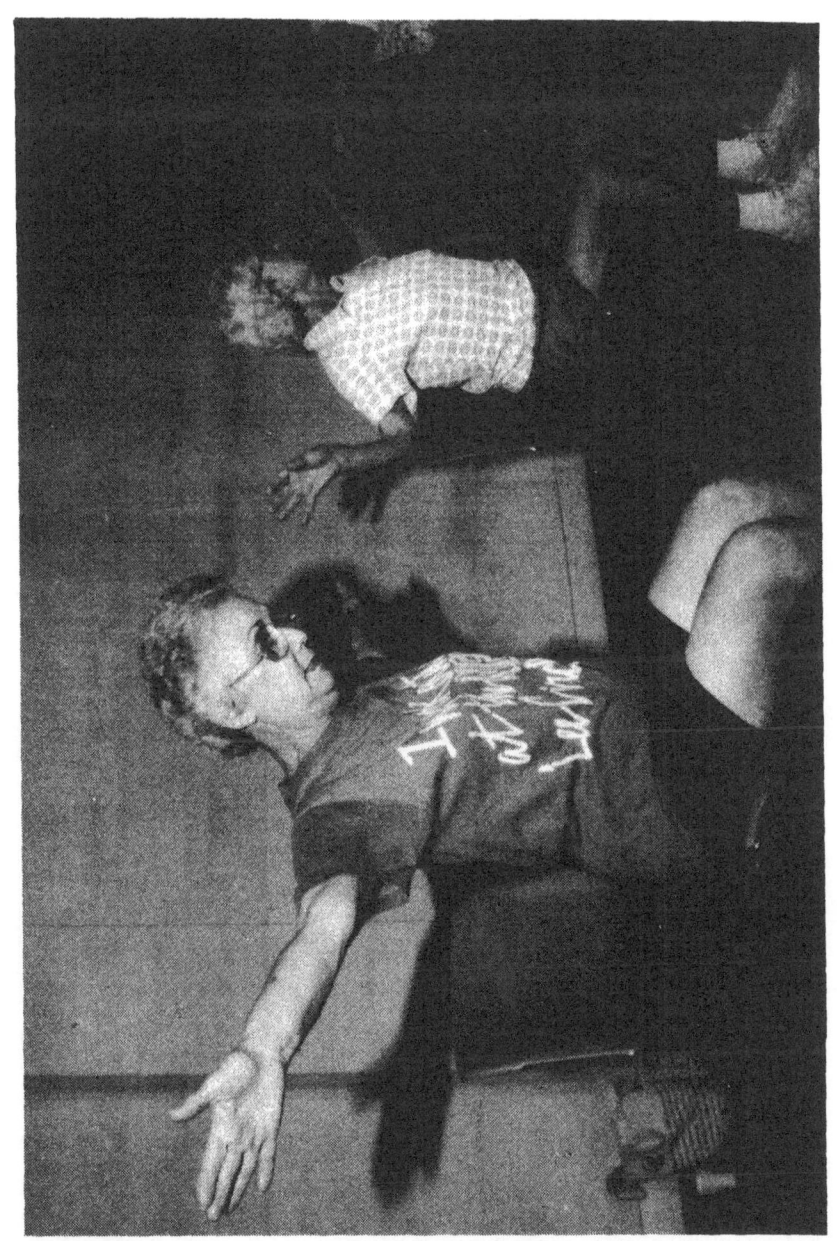

Chair exercise – arm stretch and rotation

137

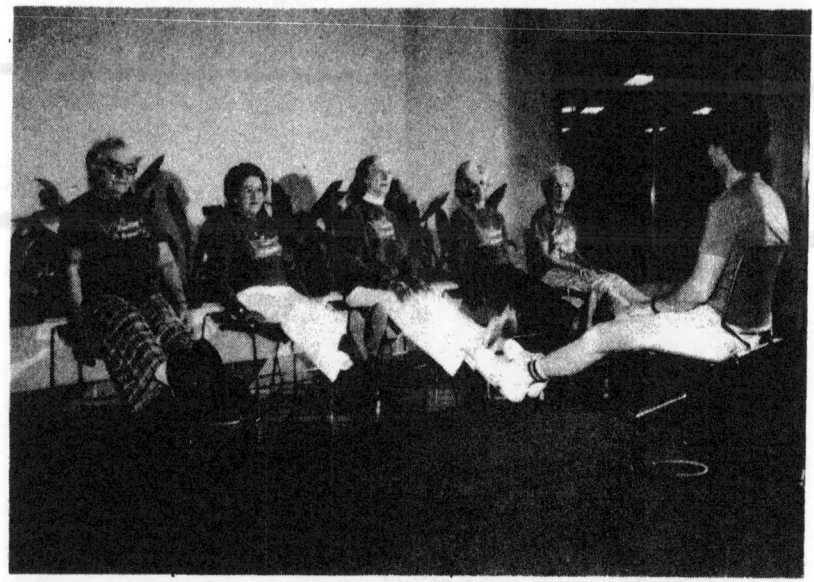

Small group exercise practice — foot rotation and flexion exercises

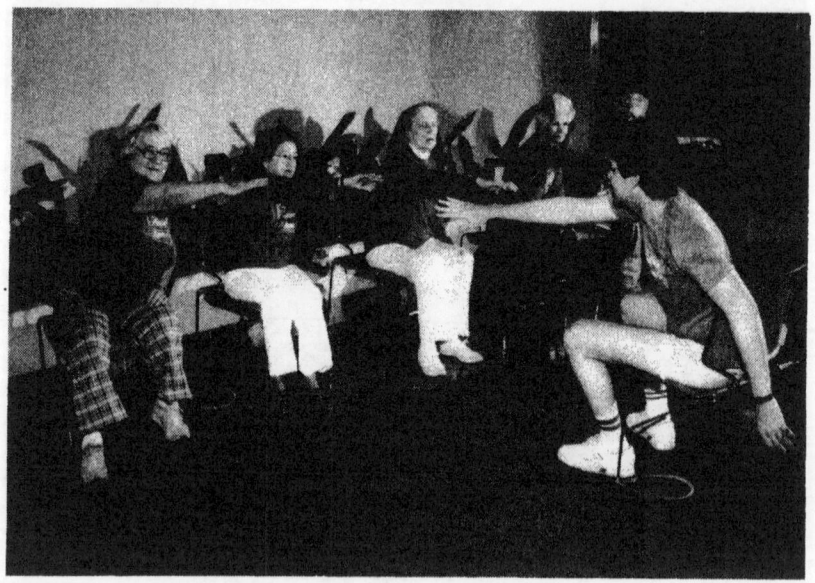

Small group exercise practice — arm stretches

- Hold arms directly in front of self, squeeze and open hands repetitively, do hand circles, shake the hands out, massage the hands, arms, shoulders, and neck.
- Lift arms to shoulder height parallel to the floor, stretch to one side and then to the other.
- Reach upward, one arm at a time, like climbing a ladder or stretching up to the sky.
- Slowly reach downward, each hand sliding down the side of a leg, then sit straight up.
- Reach downward to the right, center, and next to the left.
- Slowly pat the body with both hands starting from the head and go through the whole body to the feet.

- Rotate shoulders forward and then backward.
- Raise one shoulder at a time and then lower the shoulder.
- Raise both shoulders up, then down.

- Slowly rotate the head to the right, straight ahead, next to the left, then downward (try to place the chin on the chest), followed by slowly bringing the head up straight forward.
- Bend the head by lowering the ear to the shoulder, then slowly lower the head in the opposite direction to touch the other shoulder.
- Turn the head to look over the right shoulder and then slowly turn to look over the left shoulder.
- Rotate shoulders again.

- Raise legs parallel to the floor (participants may need to hold onto the chair) and have the feet touch at the toes and alternately at the heels.
- With legs raised have feet pointing away from the person then bend at the ankles to have them point upward toward the person.
- Next, with legs raised turn the feet at the ankles in one direction and then in the other direction.
- Raise legs and kick vigorously up and down.
- Stamp feet on floor vigorously.
- Gently massage and move (tighten and loosen) any part of the body that seems tight or aching. Take three more slow deep breaths and relax.

STANDING EXERCISES

- Slightly bending at the knees, do full arm rotations, one arm at a time, approximately ten times forward and ten times backward, keeping the arms straight as you rotate them.

- Still slightly bending at the knees, place hands on the hips and do hip rotations. Next, with the hands on the stomach and the back do pelvic movements front and backward.
- Bending at the knees, arms parallel to the floor with palms facing away from body, turn slowly to the right and then to the left. Next, make large circle with arms.
- Bending at the knees, slide the right arm down the right leg toward the foot, then slide the left arm down the left leg toward the foot.
- Next, gently and slowly reach up to the sky, like climbing a ladder. Stretching the arms, hands, and body upward.

- Lightly jog in place for a few minutes keeping the head up, shaking the hands, loosening up the body, turning slightly at the waist. A modified way of jogging is to keep the balls of the feet in contact with the floor alternately lifting the heels.

- Standing next to a chair do leg exercises, one leg at a time, approximately five to ten repetitions of each exercise.
- Hold onto the chair with left arm and kick right leg forward.
- Hold onto the chair with right arm and kick left leg forward.
- Hold onto the chair with left arm and lift right leg out to the side.
- Hold onto the chair with right arm and lift left leg out to the side.
- Hold onto the chair with left arm and make large leg circles with the right leg.
- Hold onto the chair with right arm and make large leg circles with the left leg.
- Hold onto the chair with left arm and slowly kick right leg backward.
- Hold onto the chair with the right arm and slowly kick left leg backward.
- Hold onto the chair with the left arm and slowly lift up the right leg at the knee.

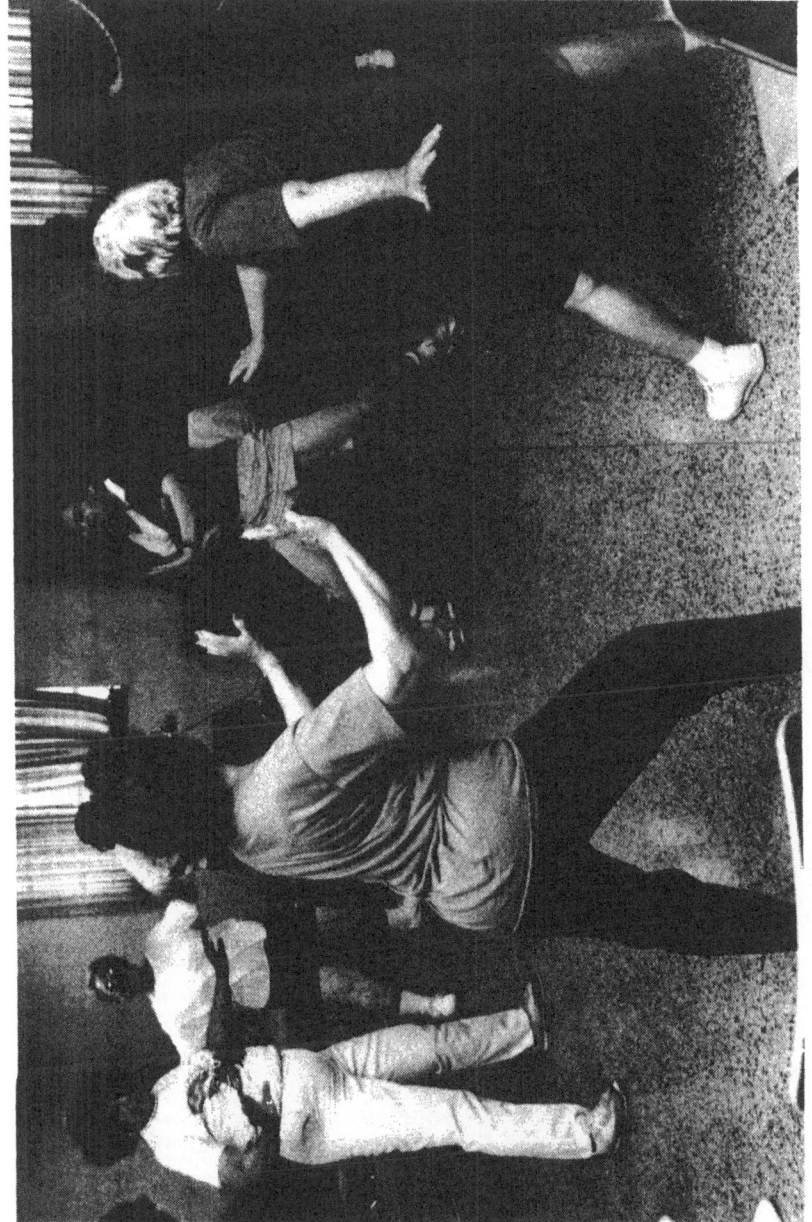

Balance and agility exercises
With knees bent, gently rotate at the waist.

141

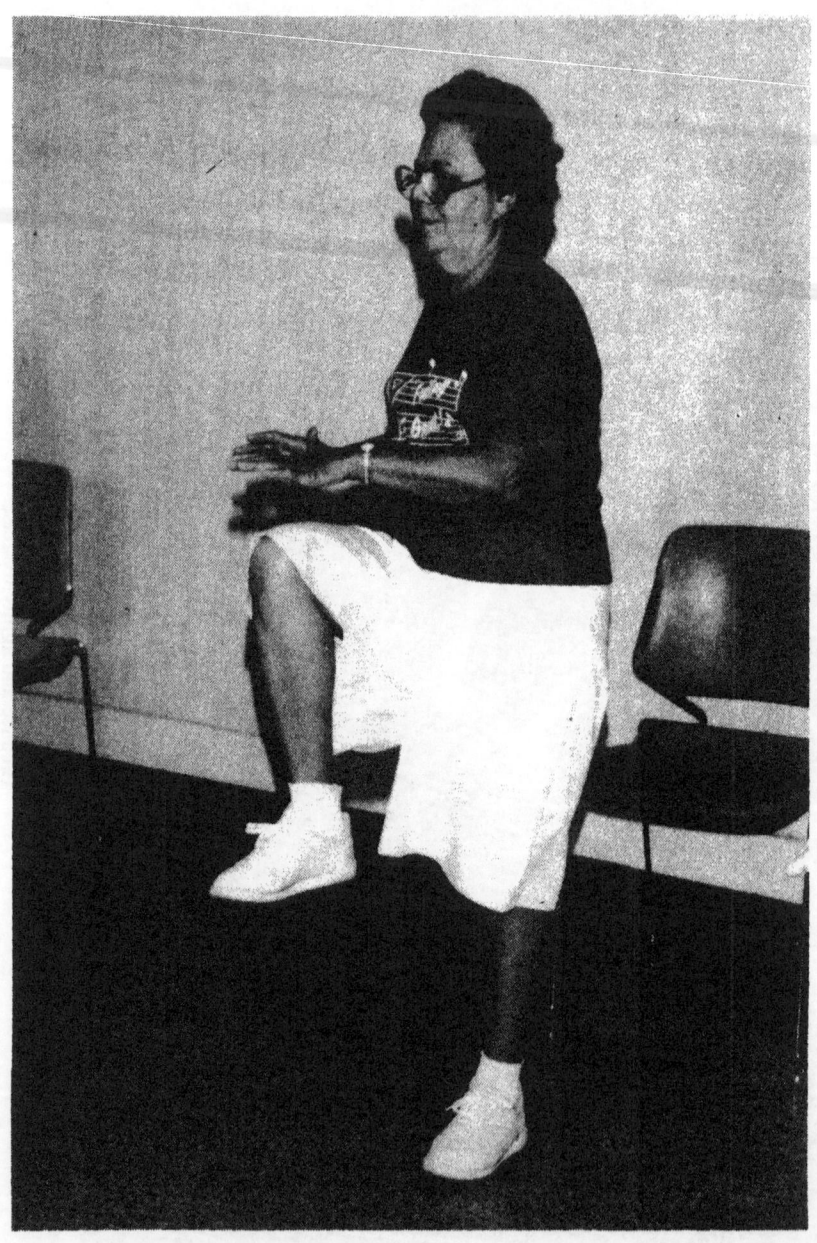

Leg lifts

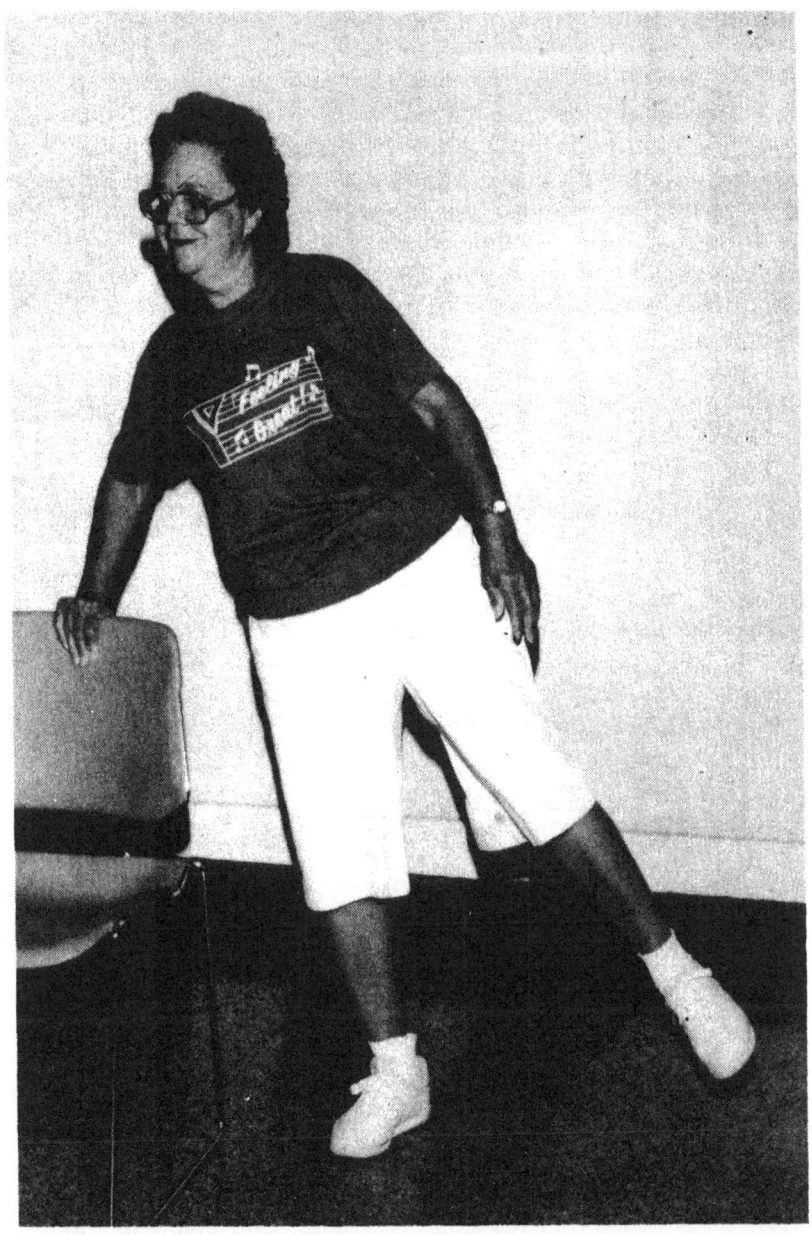

Leg lifts to the side

- Hold onto the chair with the right arm and slowly lift up the left leg at the knee.

- Next, do some loosening up by slowly jogging or walking (depending on the individual's physical condition) in place, raising the feet only a couple of inches off the floor.

- Then, standing behind the chair, slowly do slight bends and then straighten up. Do not bend down too far because participants' muscles may not be strong enough to lift them properly without hurting their backs.

WALKING (CARDIOVASCULAR EXERCISE) ROUTINE

The wearing of sturdy, well-fitting supportive walking/jogging shoes that provide a good heel and arch support should be stressed to participants.

Participants should walk in a free form fashion in a large circle. Begin walking at a normal pace and then speed it up to a brisk pace for two to five minutes. Next slow to a regular walking speed but take high steps (do this for a couple of minutes) — change to walking faster with long strides — change to skipping for a few minutes — then change to sliding side to side — finish the routine by walking as fast as possible or even jogging for about five minutes. Then have participants walk slowly to cool down while taking their target heart rate.

In this routine, the instructor should improvise with various arm movements, hip movements, leg movements, skipping and sliding side to side. The routine can be done at least two times during the exercise class. The length of time doing fast movements should be determined by the participants' abilities. Allow people who get tired to slow down and walk at a comfortable pace, while those who are in better condition to continue to briskly walk to build up their endurance.

The instructor can offer comments to sensitize and enrich the participants' awareness of the benefits of the walking activity. A few suggested comments are: "Is it more comfortable to walk fast or slow?" "Do your shoulders relax as you swing your arms?"

Brisk walking and light jogging outside the YMCA

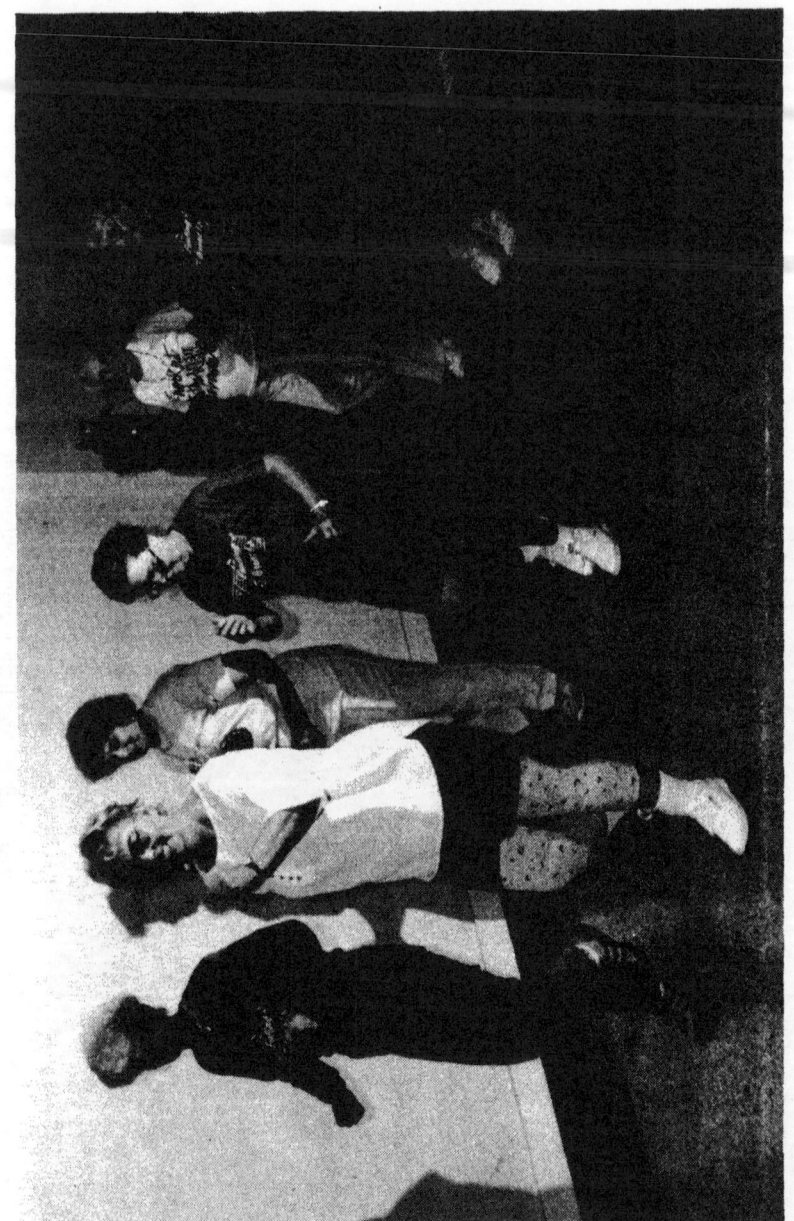

Brisk walking and light jogging

"Do any parts of the body feel tight and can you loosen them during the walk?" "Can you feel your spine straighten as you walk?" "Do you enjoy walking to music, in silence or talking while you walk?"

Walking as a Leisure Exercise

Walking is a great daily exercise because it offers similar benefits to running without the high risk of pain and injury. It is an ideal activity that people of any age or fitness level can participate in.

In brisk walking, the hands should be loosely clenched, not squeezed hard. The arm action should swing forward with the opposite leg movement. The arms work like pendulums and bending the arms at the elbows to ninety degrees shortens the pendulum and allows the person to speed up the arm strokes as he/she speeds up the steps. The elbows should be positioned close to the body and the body as a whole should be erect and as tall as possible when walking (Grey, 1985). The longer the stride the lower the individual will be to the ground, but from the waist up he/she should walk tall. For good posture, the head should always face straight ahead, not downward. Some people are afraid of walking briskly and will automatically look downward in fear of tripping over something. It may be helpful to look straight forward, a few feet in front of the person, on the ground rather than looking directly at their feet, which will strain their necks and produce bad posture.

When participants are walking with a friend it is helpful to have the friend watch their posture for feedback on their walking stance. Good posture allows the body to be more effective in its movement and feels better.

For more information the serious walker should refer to some current books on racewalking such as *Racewalk To Fitness* by Howard Jacobson and *Racewalking For Fun And Fitness* by John Gray.

Some guidelines for brisk walking exercise:

1. Warm muscles by performing slow movement, then do stretching exercises before and after walking to prevent sore muscles.
2. Start slowly and increase pace, time, and distance gradually.

3. Let heart rate, rather than miles per hour, be a guide to determining intensity.
4. Drink plenty of fluids before and after walking.
5. Do not eat for about two hours before or twenty minutes after walking.
6. To make the walk interesting, vary route and when possible walk with friends, or join a local walking group. Some shopping malls allow organized groups of senior citizens to briskly walk through the mall early in the morning before some of the stores open. Especially on rainy or cold days, this is a very enjoyable way to exercise and socialize.
7. It is not recommended to use leg weights because they put an extra strain on the joints and can throw off the individual's gait.
8. For those people who are in good physical condition, for added intensity and an upper body workout, carry light hand weights and pump arms, forward and backward, when walking.
9. As previously noted in the exercise guideline a good sturdy shoe is essential to provide proper support and to prevent injuries. Participants who are serious about brisk walking should obtain a good shoe, learn about foot care, and know about the care and wear of their shoes. For active individuals their shoes may only provide good support for about six months and then must be replaced. Wearing an expensive pair of shoes that are worn out can give a person serious foot problems.

Benefits of the Walking Exercise:
1. increases efficiency of heart and lungs
2. improves circulation
3. lowers the resting heart rate
4. lowers blood pressure
5. improves endurance and stamina
6. tones the leg muscles
7. helps improve flexibility
8. improves stability, agility and balance
9. burns calories

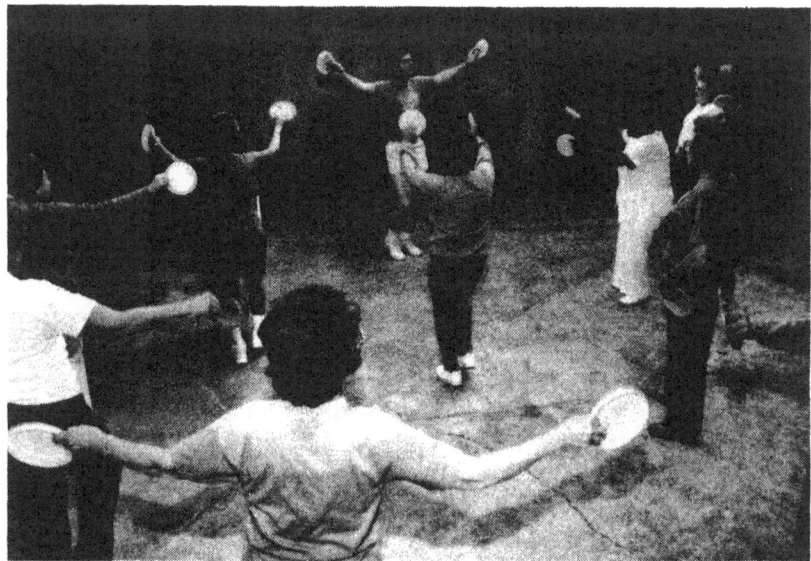

Frisbee exercise – arm circles
With arms out the side, make small and large circles rotating at the shoulder.

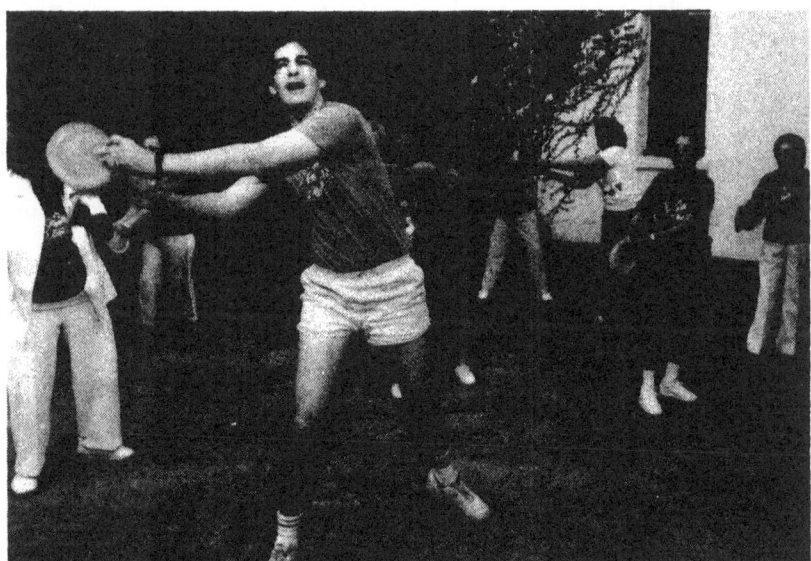

Frisbee exercise
Stretch arms to the left and snap frisbees, to the center and snap frisbees, to the right and snap frisbees, over the head and snap frisbees, and then at knee level and snap frisbees. Continue repetitions of the pattern.

BROOMSTICK EXERCISES

Apparatus: broomstick

Activities: Hold the broomstick with two hands spread apart, keeping the arms straight.

- Slowly lift the broomstick horizontally over the head ten times.
- Lift the broomstick horizontally and place behind the head resting on the neck; turn at the waist.
- From the chest, push out the broomstick horizontally ten times.
- Hold the broomstick horizontally at shoulder level directly in front, twist left arm all the way to the right and then twist right arm to the left, crossing the arms.
- Hold the broomstick out horizontally with both arms wide apart and gently swing it from side to side.
- Hold the broomstick horizontally over your head and raise one arm while lowering the other, stretching at the side.
- Hold the ends of the broomstick with each hand and while bending at the knees, keeping the back straight, touch the right foot and then the left foot.
- Hold the ends of the broomstick and walk with the fingers in and back out on the stick.
- Throw the broomstick from hand to hand, back and forth.
- Improvise with other good exercises that can be done with a broomstick.
- While performing some of the simpler exercises with the broomstick, participants can lightly jog to music.

Benefits:
1. exercises trunk and shoulder muscles
2. increases range of motion while exercising both sides of the body
3. cardiovascular endurance exercise, especially when jogging while exercising

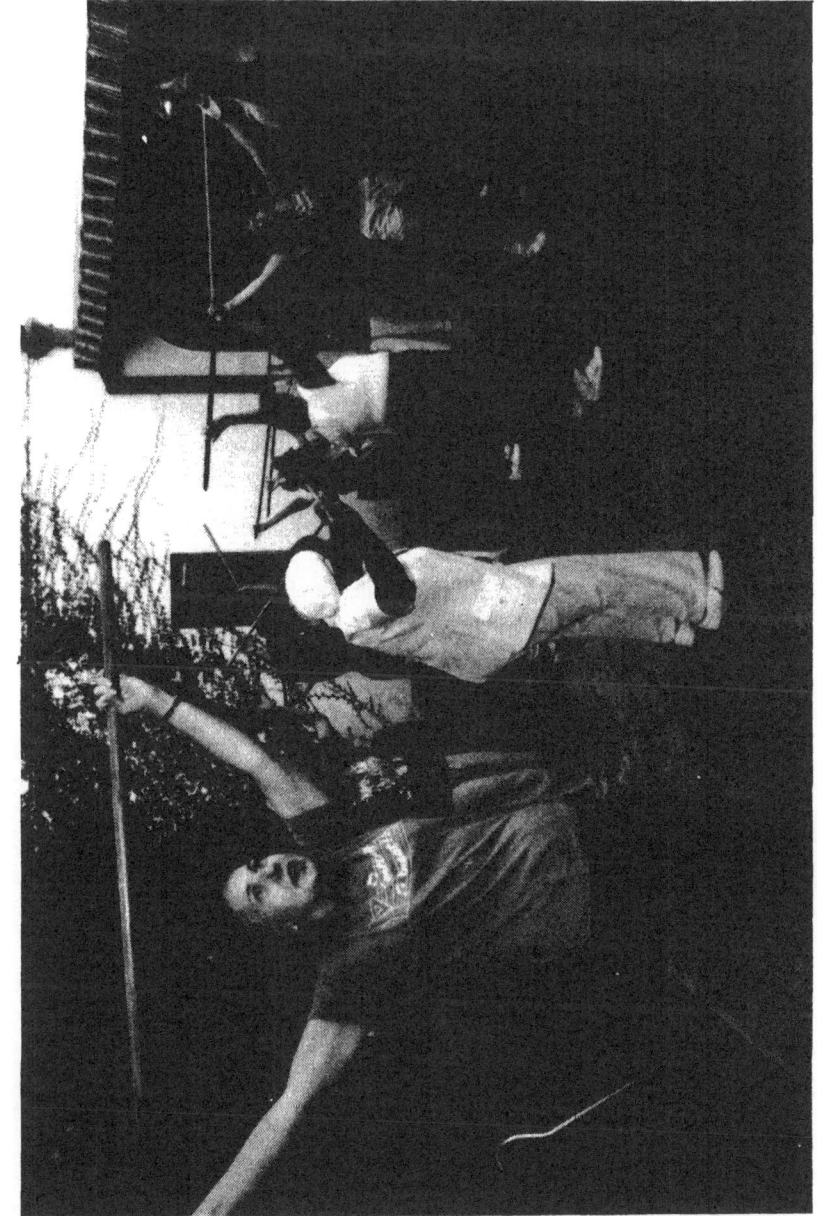

Broomstick exercises done on the patio of the YMCA
Raise broomstick over the head and twist at the waist.

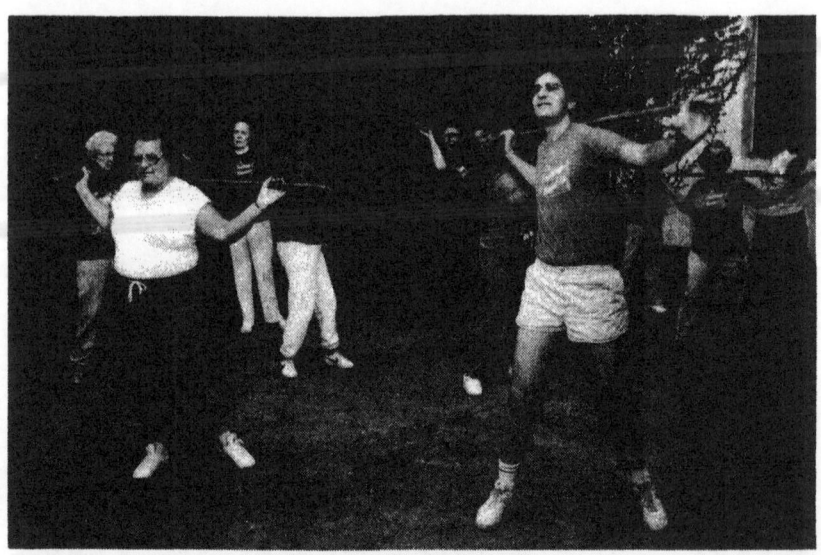

Broomstick exercises

Hold broomstick at either end and place on the shoulders. Keep knees and limbs flexed, feet apart, and heels firm on the ground. Then turn at the waist to the right and to the left.

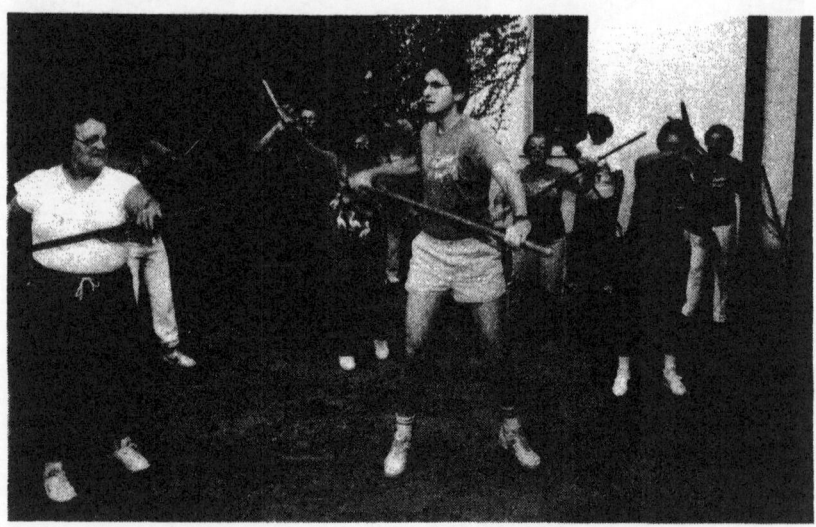

Broomstick exercise — swimming arm movements with broomstick

RUBBER TUBING EXERCISES

Apparatus: rubber tubing (approximately one half inch width, 1/16 inch thick, and 16 inches long). The tubing can be purchased at a medical supplies store.

Tie knots at either end of the tubing so it is easy to hold on the insides of the knots and gives participants greater control of the tubing. Make sure that the knots are tied tightly and there are no tears in the tubing.

An exercise rubber band, 3/8 inch thick, can also be used for these exercises. Two books which describe the rubber band exercises are, *The Rubber Band Shape-Up Program* by Kyle and Sandy Zook and *Tamilee Webb's Original Rubber Band Workout* by Tamilee Webb.

Activities: to be done five to ten times for each exercise. Do various stretching, range of motion, and flexibility exercises with the apparatus. These exercises can be done sitting in a chair, standing, or some can possibly be done while lightly jogging.

- Hold the rubber tubing (with each hand at the end of the tube) above your head and pull to the sides.
- Hold the tubing at chest level and pull to the sides.
- Hold the tubing at the waist level and pull to the sides.
- Hold the tubing at shoulder height, left arm outstretched and pulling with the right arm. Next reverse the activity with right arm outstretched and pulling with the left arm.
- Step on the tubing so the knot is on the inside of your foot and pull the other end of the tube upward by the side of the leg. Do this activity on both sides of the body.
- Sitting in a chair, hold the tubing at both ends, put one foot in the middle of the tube and push against the tube; after a few repetitions then switch to the other foot. Another activity is to keep your leg pushed against the tube and pull on the tubing, exercising your arms.

Benefits:
1. Strengthens the arm, shoulder, and back muscles.

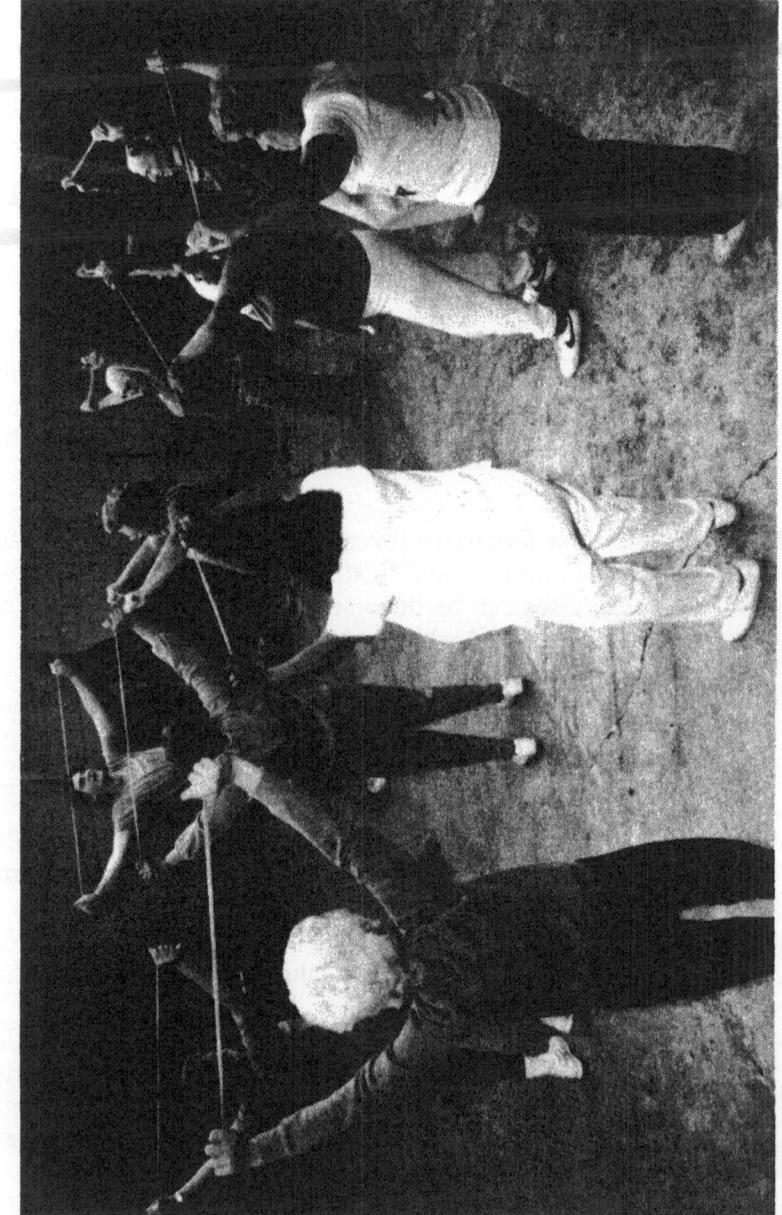

Rubber tubing exercise done on the patio of the YMCA — rubber tubing stretch for upper arm strength

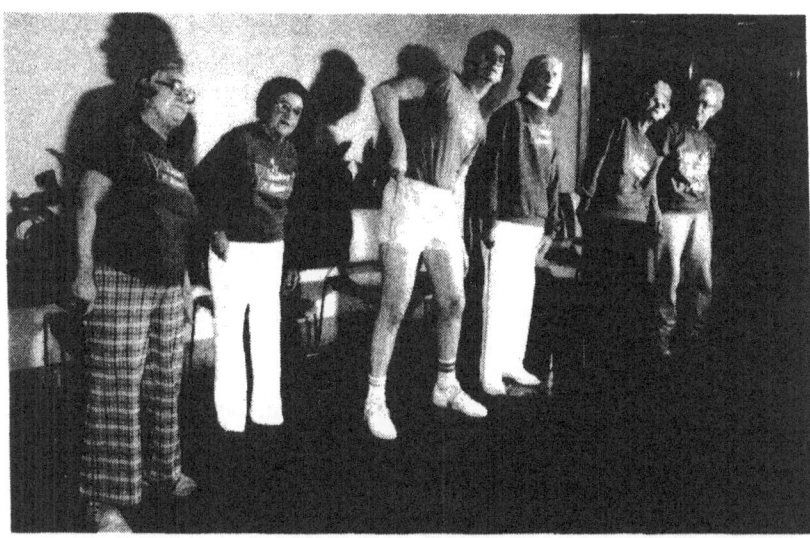

Small group exercise practice
Hold rubber tubing under foot with knot at the end of the tubing on the inside of the shoe. Pull up at the side.

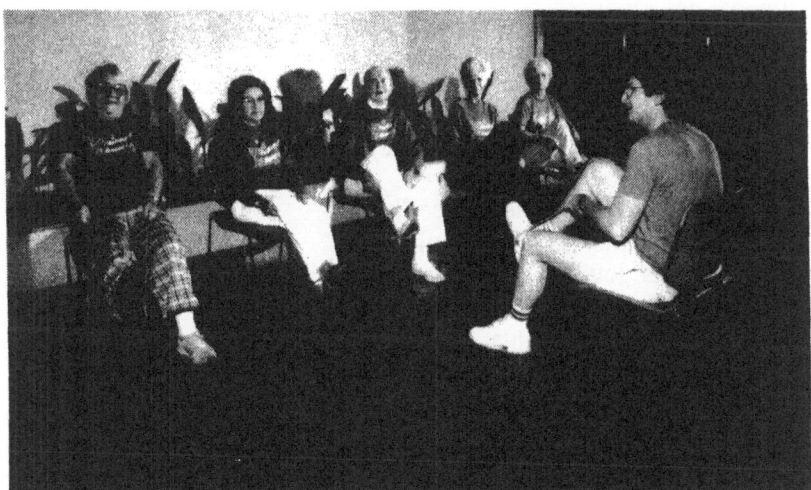

Small group exercise practice
While seated, with both hands hold rubber tubing firmly under foot. Pull up with arms and stretch rubber tubing upward for ten repetitions. Then hold the tubing firmly in hand and push foot out, stretching the rubber tubing for ten repetitions.

2. Increases muscle strength and endurance of the shoulder girdle, upper arms, torso, lower back, thighs, waist, hands, and abdomen muscles.

HAND-WEIGHT EXERCISES

Apparatus: light two pound hand-weights or soft wrist-weights. Light weights can be purchased which will strap or attach to the wrist. These are especially helpful for people who cannot hold weights due to arthritic fingers and hands.

Activities; Sitting in a chair or standing do various lifting, full range of motion, stretching, and strengthening exercises with light weights. These exercises should be done slowly without any jerking movements. Fast action jerking movements could result in a torn muscle. Participants should not hold their breath while exercising, but be able to breathe and talk comfortably in the activity. Make sure participants do not strain themselves by overexerting past a comfortable level of exercise. It is recommended not to jog while lifting the hand-weights unless participants are in good physical condition and have built up enough strength to do the exercise easily. Jogging while lifting weights puts extra strain on the heart.

Hold weights in either arm, keep legs slightly bent for balance.

• Push the weights up to the ceiling.
• Push out to the front and to the sides.
• Hang arms downward and pull up by one side at a time.
• Hang arms downward and slide down one leg at a time.
• Punch out with weights.
• Curl up from elbow to shoulder.
• Curl from the sides to the center.
• Turn at the wrists, making large arm circles.

Benefits:
1. upper arm and torso strengthening
2. endurance exercise
3. upper body toning exercise

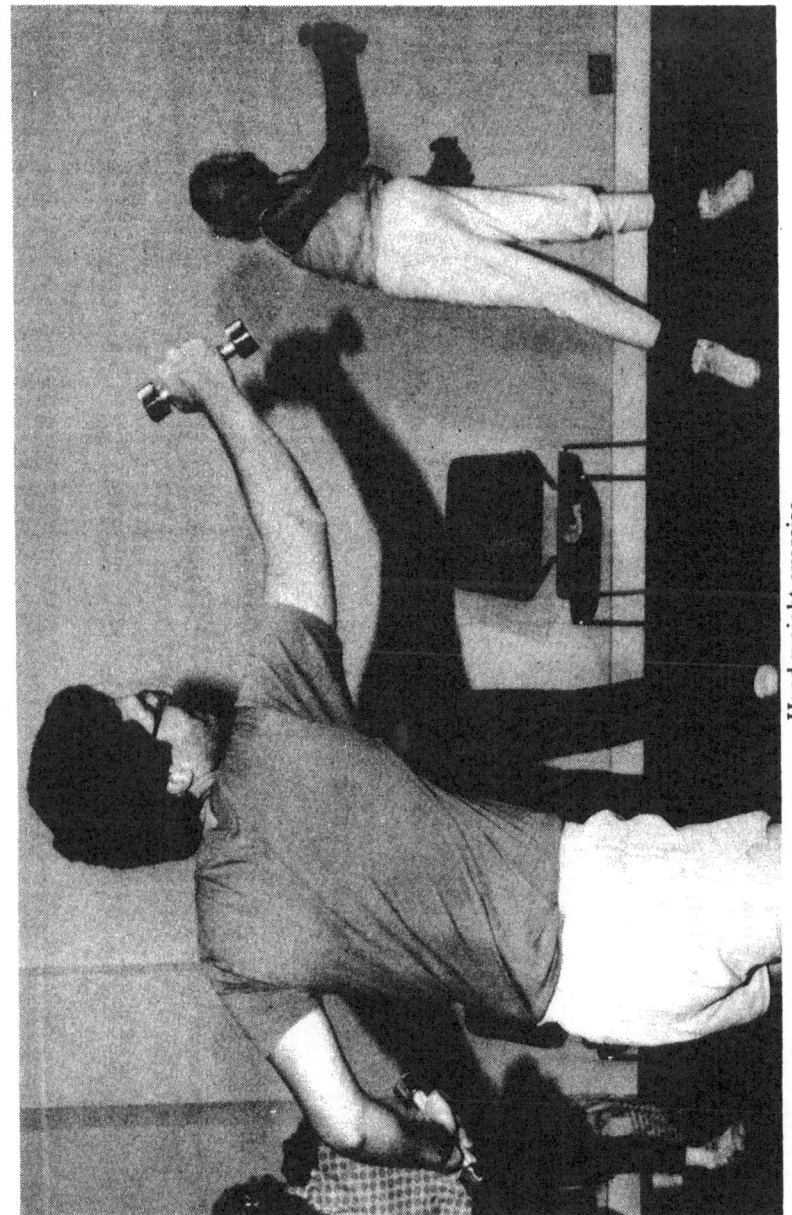

Hand-weight exercise

Stretch arm forward, then back (slightly bending at the knees and turning at the waist).

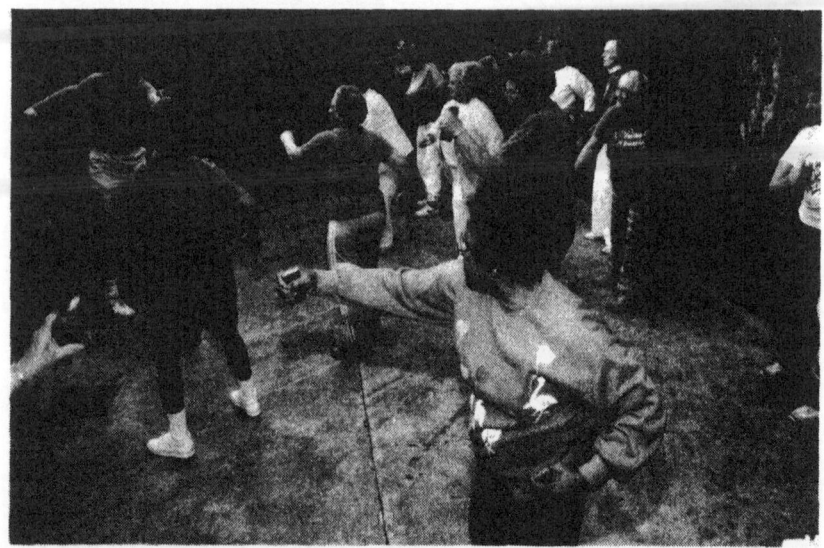

Hand-weight exercises done on the patio of the YMCA
Stretch arm to the front and side then back (slightly bending at the knees and turning at the waist).

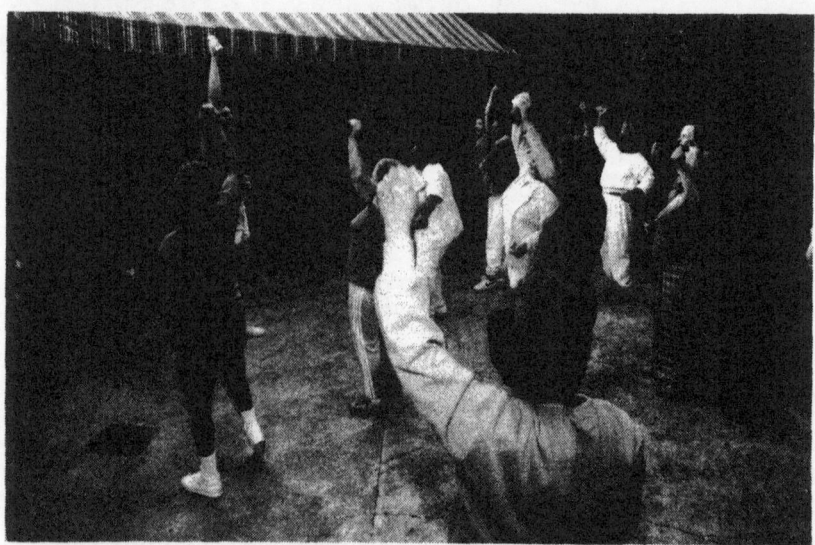

Hand-weight exercise
Stretch upward with the hand-weights for upper arm strengthening. People who are in good physical condition may want to lightly jog while exercising with light hand-weights.

MAT EXERCISES

Teach participants the correct way to get down onto a mat and how to get back up. In doing various mat exercises make sure participants are careful not to strain their back. Begin with repetitions of five times. Over time, work toward repetitions of ten times or more. Have participants do only as much as they feel comfortable. For a comprehensive program see *The Y's Way To A Healthy Back* by Alexander Melleby, New Century Publishers, New Jersey, 1982. The suggested mat exercises are also explained in the book, *The Official YMCA Fitness Program*.

Some suggested mat exercises are as follows.

- seated stretches
- single and double knee flex
- single leg raises
- stretch leg-overs
- bicycling on your back
- sit ups with knees bent
- "the cat"
- knee-to-nose and kick-back
- abdominal pump/pelvic lift
- chest stretch on the mat

This is also a good time to take advantage of some relaxation exercises while lying on the mat. See page 167 for more information on relaxation exercises.

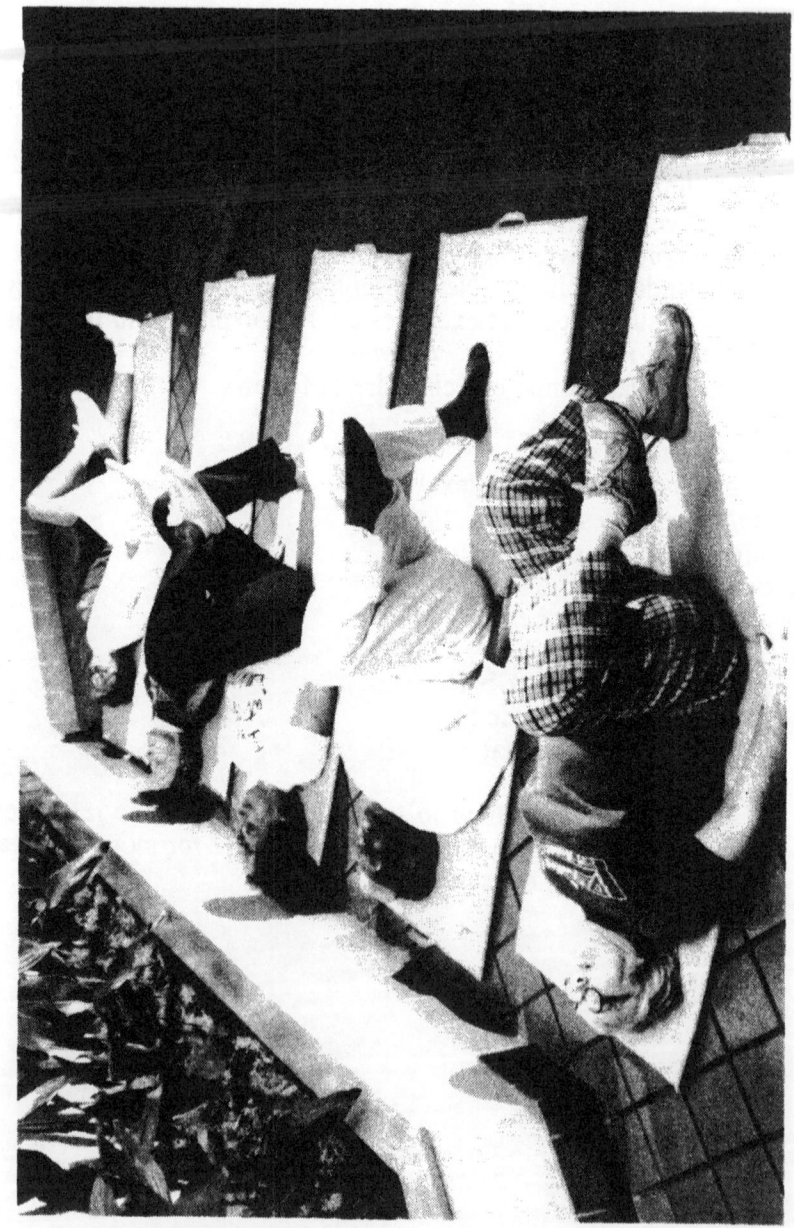

Mat exercise — knee lifts

While lying on the back, arms to the side with knees raised and feet flat on mat, slowly bring one knee at a time up to the chest and then down.

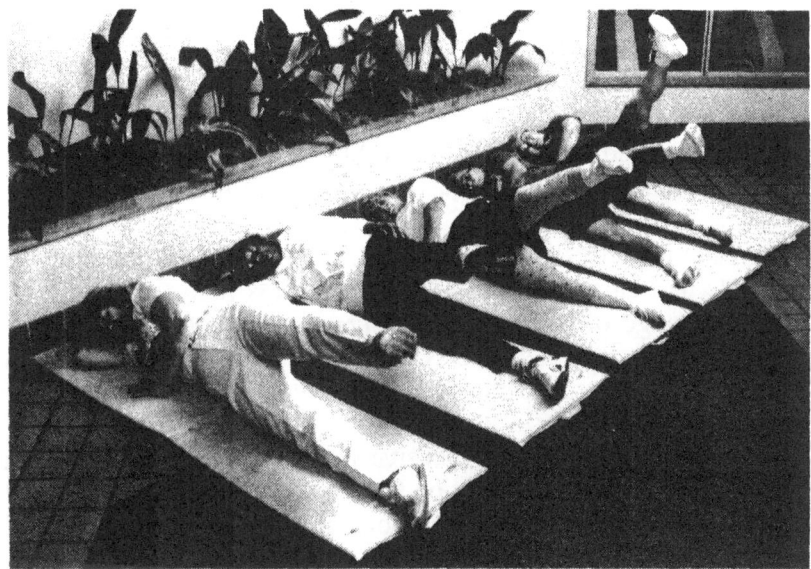

Mat exercise — leg lifts

While lying on the side, fully extended with legs straight, head resting on the arm, slowly raise one leg, then lower.

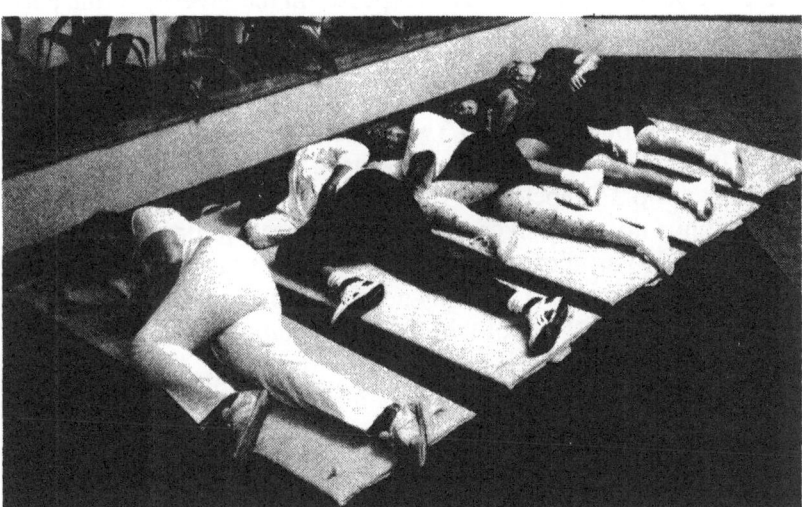

Mat exercise — leg slide

Lying on the side, one arm resting under the head, gently slide the top leg toward the shoulder and then slowly slide it back. Breathe slowly and deeply while performing the exercise activity. This exercise can help relax the muscles in the lower back and reduce lower back tension.

SWIMMING AND WATER EXERCISES

A multipurpose program designed to increase cardiovascular endurance, flexibility, and muscle endurance. Swimmers and non-swimmers find aquatics an enjoyable method of exercising safely without fear of falling or sustaining injuries that occur outside of water.

Water exercises take the weight off of weight-bearing joints and enable participants to move freely with less joint pain and with a greater range of motion (especially aiding those individuals who have arthritis and osteoporosis). For many participants, overcoming the fear of water is a major hurdle which they can work toward slowly.

For an excellent comprehensive water exercise program contact your local Arthritis Foundation for the nearest "Arthritis — Aquatic Program." This program was developed in conjunction with the YMCA and is held at YMCAs around the country.

Activities: Recommended length of the class session is approximately 30 to 45 minutes. This depends on the severity of the participants' arthritis, the tolerance of participants, the length of time it takes to get into the water and adjusted, and other variables. Classes should begin with 5 minutes of limbering up exercises in the water. Exercises should start with 3 repetitions and gradually progress to 8 to 10 repetitions. The more advanced participant may slowly increase up to 15 repetitions of an exercise. If a person experiences pain while doing the exercises, it may be best to limit the amount of repetitions. Participants should use their full range of motion while doing the exercises. They may need to stable themselves by holding onto the side of the pool while they do some of the exercises.

1. Flexibility and balance

• leg lifts — front, side, back
• knee lifts
• knee bends
• walking, marching
• arm exercises

• wrist and finger exercises
• stretching at the waist

2. Cardiovascular movements

• briskly walking, bicycle pedaling, hopping, running in place, twists with constant movement using arms and legs.
• breathing exercises—bubble breathing, blowing to expand lung capacity

3. Swimming and floating using kick boards and learning how to swim; or performing nonswimming activities in the water such as water basketball or pushing balls under water to create resistance for strengthening activity.

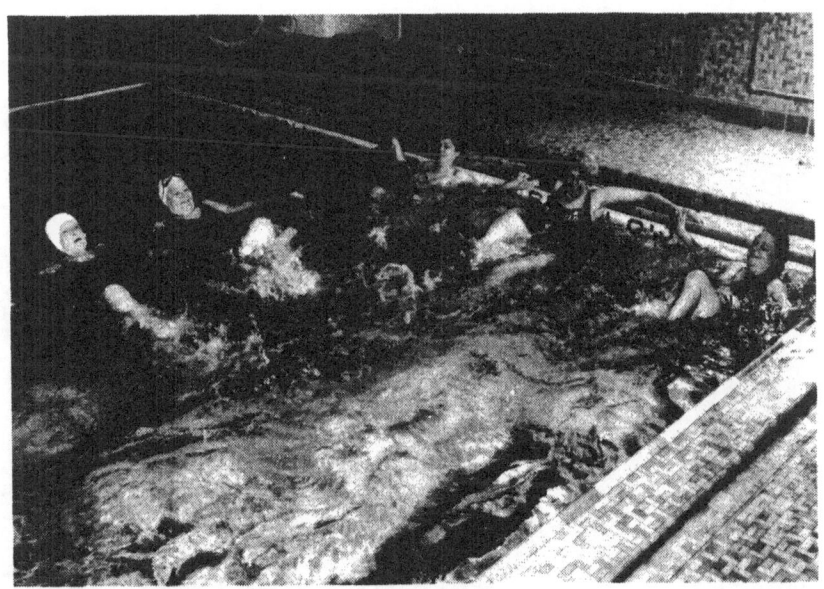

Water exercise

ACTIVE GAMES

Goal: Group activity for fun peer group interaction and exercise. Competitive and noncompetitive games that everyone can plan, anyone can win, and people can practice to develop their skills without fear of failure.

Activities:
1. various circle games, some games using light-weight balls
2. relay races, some races using props for more fun
3. adapted basketball and other sport activities
4. "New Games" activities taken from the book *The New Games*, edited by Andrew Fluegelman, A Headlands Press Book, 1974.
5. Play some of the participants' favorite pastime games and have participants make up new games.

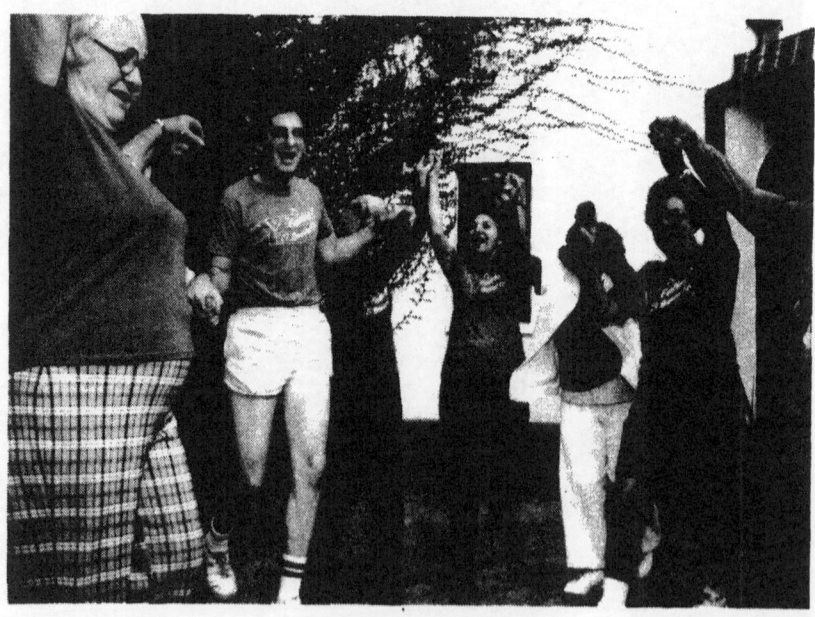

Having fun on the patio

Benefits:
1. develops coordination
2. develops agility and balance
3. promotes enjoyable group interaction
4. offers participants games they enjoy playing, a way to relax and exercise
5. develops friendships

RELAXATION EXERCISES

In the second part of the program after the mat exercises or games, the instructor may want to end the "Feeling Great!" session with a relaxation period. But keep in mind that some participants may not want to join in relaxation exercises because the activity can make them very deeply relaxed and very possibly put them to sleep. Or possibly they may feel uneasy with the eyes closed, sitting or lying down silently, in a room full of people. But, many participants may be looking for a way to deeply relax, an activity which on their own they may have much difficulty in achieving, resulting in poor sleeping patterns.

Just as exercise is important to keep the body in shape, relaxation helps to rejuvenate the whole being through quieting the mind and body, relaxing the breathing, and resting the muscles of the body. Proper relaxation is as important as exercising because if the body does not relax from stress and tension, it will become ill. All exercise programs include the tensing and relaxing of muscles but the deep relaxation technique further calms the body and mind.

Relaxation aids in sleeping, coping with stress, lowering blood pressure, and in gaining clarity of mind. Three major components of relaxation are deep breathing, visualization, and progressive muscle relaxation. These components can be effective when done separately or in combination with each other.

Deep abdominal breathing—Participants can be sitting, standing, or lying on a mat while they take slow, full, deep breaths, inhaling gently through their nose from their lower stomachs. As they are doing this exercise, a good image for them to focus on is to imagine that they are breathing from their feet and the breath is traveling throughout their whole body and finally being released through their hands. As they inhale, they should imagine taking in good, clean, refreshing air, and as they breathe out they are breathing out their tiredness and pains, breathing in joy and wellness.

Steps to abdominal breathing:

1. Place hands (fingers spread) on abdomen.
2. Breathe through your nose.
3. Abdomen should rise with each inhalation.
4. Abdomen should fall (or lower) with each exhalation.
5. Chest should move in harmony with the abdomen.
6. Scan body for tension, especially forehead, upper back/neck, jaw/teeth.
7. Think about "letting go" of muscle tension as you continue with your abdominal breathing.
8. You may want to start by counting your inhalations.

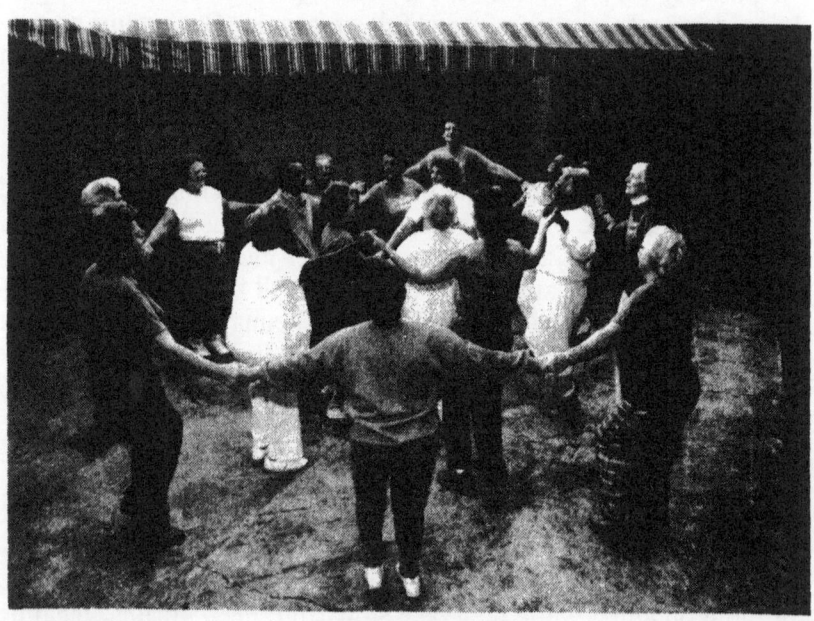

Group games

Visualization — Participants can be sitting or lying down, breathing in a relaxed manner, and imagining a pleasant scene, memory, or person. The instructor should talk the participants through the visualization and then let them be with the image for about five minutes, deeply relaxing.

Progressive muscle relaxation — Participants can be sitting in a chair or lying down. Have participants focus on a part of their body, tense it, and then relax it, going from head to toe, tensing and relaxing the different parts of the whole body. While participants are doing this process, ask them to deeply breathe in a relaxing manner which can help in releasing tension.

Recommended relaxation suggestions for participants to do at home or at work are sitting or standing static stretching; being in a quiet room, listening to some relaxing music and practicing visualization with pleasant imagery; taking a short walk; and closing the eyes and practicing abdominal breathing. It is recommended to take a relaxation break daily. It also feels good to incorporate a relaxation phase after the exercise work-out (after cool-down).

Guided relaxation requires a soft tone of voice and a willingness to pace the exercise slowly. There are numerous good publications on relaxation techniques and these techniques are also often taught in yoga classes. I encourage interested instructors to practice the relaxation techniques so they can personally experience deep relaxation and be able to easily guide participants in the activity.

Chapter VI

Program Materials

DESCRIPTION OF FORMS

A. *Health History Appraisal Form* and *Physical Activity Profile*, page 174.
B. *Personal Fitness Progress Chart* and *Fitness Log*, page 178.
C. *Goals, Homework, Periodic Review*, page 180.
D. *Contract/Goals Form*, page 181.
E. *Program Evaluation* and *Recommendation Form*, page 182.
F. *Attendance Form*, page 183.
G. *Program Statistics*, page 184.
H. *"Feeling Great!"* brochure and *"Welcome To The 'Feeling Great!' Program"* guide, page 186.
I. *Participant Phone Number Directory* (not shown)

****

A. *Health History Appraisal Form* and *Physical Activity Profile*, page 174

This form is a good fitness profile which gives background information about each participant. Participants are not required to see a doctor before beginning the program unless they have serious physical ailments, a heart condition or high blood pressure. It is recommended that all participants tell their doctor that they are joining an exercise program and ask if they should be cautious of performing any particular exercise.
The noted YMCA forms have been adjusted to reflect the profile of older adult participants.

B. *Personal Fitness Progress Chart* and *Fitness Log*, page 178

The "Progress Chart" is for recording basic information such as name, age, date, height, weight, target heart rate, maximum heart rate, blood pressure, and pulse. This form will enable participants to monitor their physical changes and keep abreast of their progress. The "Fitness Log" gives participants an easy monthly check on how often they have been exercising.

C. *Goals, Homework, Periodic Review*, page 180

Once participants have made a commitment to attend the program they should develop their goals. The rationale for setting goals is to help participants decide what they want to achieve in the "Feeling Great!" program and to help them stay focused on reaching their goals. Once realistic goals are set, the instructor should provide a daily exercise homework schedule including the exercise pattern, length of time to exercise, diet suggestions, and motivational key points. A periodic review of the homework should be done every three or four weeks and, if needed, adjustments made.

Let the class know about some of the participants' exercise plans and positive changes experienced so they can support each other in their efforts.

D. *Contract/Goals Form*, page 181

This form is used to help participants focus on their short- and long-range goals and assist them with making a clear, firm agreement with themselves and their instructor on their exercise/diet activity.

E. *Program Evaluation* and *Recommendation Form*, page 182

It is recommended that participants formally evaluate the program and provide their ideas and suggestions every month or whenever deemed appropriate by the instructor or class. Also, Recommendation Forms should be available to participants at all classes for those people who would rather write down their suggestions than verbally discuss them. Participants can take these forms home and jot down suggestions when they think of them. For some participants it is easier to give feedback by writing their thoughts down, rather than having to confront someone personally.

F. *Attendance Form*, page 183

This form aids in keeping good records and noting when participants are absent so the instructor or a volunteer could call them for a personal invitation/reminder to attend the class.

G. *Program Statistics, Monthly and Per Class*, page 184

It is important to record the class attendance and the fees collected in order to reflect the growth of the program. These statistics help to point out drops or gains in class attendance. A monthly chart is used to compare the seasonal class record and a rotating four week chart is used to cite each class's attendance and fees collected.

Please note that the "Feeling Great!" class is free to YMCA members, so the noted collected fees do not reflect an accurate account. Some people join the YMCA just for the "Feeling Great!" program. Therefore, their dues should be counted as a part of the collected fees when budgeting for the program.

H. *Welcome to the "Feeling Great!" Program* guide and the *"Feeling Great!"* brochure, page 186

"Welcome To The 'Feeling Great!' Program" guide provides an in-depth description of the program with answers to some of the most commonly asked questions for prospective participants.

The "Feeling Great!" brochure is a good marketing and publicity tool to advertise the program. The brochure lists the basic information on the program and also includes a registration/consent form. When joining the program it is important that all participants sign the registration/consent form to formally acknowledge their personal responsibility to their health.

I. *Participant Phone Number Directory*, (not shown)

An updated list of participants' phone numbers is given out periodically. Participants are encouraged to call and see each other between classes. This form is not listed.

YMCA OF GREATER NEW ORLEANS

HEALTH HISTORY APPRAISAL FORM

PLEASE PRINT   DATE _____

NAME _____ AGE _____

PHONE NUMBER (home) _____ (work) _____

PHYSICIAN'S NAME   _____

ADDRESS   _____

PHONE NUMBER   _____

HOSPITAL   _____

••• I choose not to fill out this Health History Appraisal Form •••

NAME_____   SIGNATURE_____

DATE_____

As requested by the exercise instructor, I have informed my physician that I am beginning an exercise program at the Lee Circle YMCA to improve my level of fitness

Signature _____

Date _____

• • • • • • • • •

1.   When was your last medical exam by your physician?   Month/Year _____

2.   YES   NO   A. Any major illness or operation in the past?

B. If yes, please specify : _____

3.   YES   NO   A. Do you exercise?
( ) Walking   ( ) Bowling
( ) Jogging   ( ) Competitive Athletics
( ) Golfing   ( ) Non-competitive Athletics
( ) Swimming   ( ) Other : _____
( ) Calisthenics

B. How would you classify your exercise pattern?
( ) Moderate & Irregular   ( ) Substantial & Regular
( ) Moderate & Regular   ( ) Physically Inactive

C. How many time a week do you exercise?   _____

YES   NO   D. Do you feel limited in any activities you do?

E. Is this due to:
( ) Breathing   ( ) Chest Pain
( ) Arm Pain   ( ) Neck Pain
( ) Back Pain   ( ) Other : _____

4. YES   NO   A. Do you smoke? ( ) Cigarettes   ( ) Cigars   ( ) Pipe

    YES   NO   B. Did you ever smoke?
                  ( ) How many years/weeks ago did you stop?   _____
                  ( ) What was the reason for discontinuing?   _____
                  ( ) How many packs per day did you smoke?   _____
                  ( ) How many years did you smoked at this level?   _____

5. YES   NO   A. Do you have diabetes or a diabetic tendency?

6. YES   NO   A. Have you ever had high blood pressure?

7. YES   NO   A. Did you ever have a heart murmur?

8. YES   NO   A. Is there a history of heart trouble in you family?

9. YES   NO   A. Is/was your cholesterol elevated?

10. YES   NO   A. Do you have palpations, skipped beats or an awareness of your heart?

11. YES   NO   A. Do you have fainting spells?

12. YES   NO   A. Are you having chest, neck, or arm pains?

    YES   NO   B. Is the pain related to any physical activity?

13. YES   NO   A. Have you ever been told of having a heart attack or heart trouble?

14. YES   NO   A. Are you taking any medication?

               B. If yes, what kind are you taking? _____
                  (dosage and frequency) _____

15. YES   NO   A. Any muscle injuries or illness now or in the past?

               B. If yes, please specify : _____

16. YES   NO   A. Any bone or joint (including spine) injuries or illness now or in the past?

               B. If yes, please specify : _____

17. YES   NO   A. Do any previous or old bone or joint injuries appear when you engage in
                  physical activities?

               B. If yes, please specify : _____

18. YES   NO   A. Weight gain in past ten years?

               B. Weight at age 40 _____   70 _____

                                 50 _____   80 _____

                                 60 _____   90 _____

               C. Present weight :   _____

               C. Present height :   _____

Y's Way To Physical Fitness

PHYSICAL ACTIVITY PROFILE

NAME _____ DATE _____

Please answer the following questions about your job and non-job related physical activity.

1. WHAT TYPE OF WORK DO YOU DO?

   _____

2. IN WHAT KIND OF BUSINESS OR INDUSTRY DO YOU WORK OR WHAT ARE YOUR HOBBIES?

   _____

3. ON THE AVERAGE DURING THE PAST YEAR, HOW MANY HOURS PER DAY HAVE YOU SPENT PERFORMING THE FOLLOWING ACTIVITIES?

Activity	*Hours per day*
Sitting, e.g. typing, writing, reading, television, etc. (not including driving)	_____
Driving auto, truck, bus, or other equipment	_____
Standing	_____
Walking	_____
Light physical labor	_____
Moderate physical labor	_____
Heavy physical labor, e.g., lifting or carrying heavy objects, digging, chopping wood	_____
Other, Specify : _____	_____

4. HOW WOULD YOU RATE THE AMOUNT OF PHYSICAL ACTIVITY YOU PERFORM IN YOUR DAILY ACTIVITIES?

   very little   little   moderate   active   very active

5. HOW WOULD YOU RATE THE AMOUNT OF PHYSICAL ACTIVITY YOU PERFORM DURING LEISURE TIME?

   very little   little   moderate   active   very active

6. ARE YOU PRESENTLY PERFORMING ANY STANDARD "PHYSICAL FITNESS" PROGRAM?

   YES _____ NO _____ If Yes, which ones? _____

7. HOW PHYSICALLY FIT DO YOU FEEL AT THE PRESENT?

   unfit   below average   average   above average   very fit

8. PROVIDING THE EQUIPMENT AND FACILITIES WERE AVAILABLE, IN WHICH PHYSICAL ACTIVITIES WOULD YOU BE INTERESTED IN LEARNING AND PARTICIPATING? PLEASE CHECK OR LIST ACTIVITIES.

Hiking	_____	Tennis	_____	Calisthenics	_____
Jogging	_____	Handball	_____	Weight Training	_____
Bicycling	_____	Volleyball	_____	Golf	_____
Swimming	_____	Badminton	_____	Supervised	
Brisk		Bowling	_____	conditioning	
Walking	_____	Gardening	_____	program	_____

   Other (Specify)

   _____

   _____

   _____

   _____

9. DO YOU HAVE ANY EXERCISE EQUIPMENT OR DEVICE AT HOME?

   YES _____ NO _____ If Yes, please specify _____

PERSONAL FITNESS PROGRESS CHART

NAME _____ AGE _____

DATE _____ WT ____ HT ____

M.H.R. _____ T.H.R. _____

TEST T-1 _____ T-2 _____ T-3 _____

MEASUREMENTS
NECK _____
ARMS _____
CHEST _____
WAIST _____
HIPS _____
THIGHS _____
CALF _____

LEE CIRCLE YMCA
936 ST. CHARLES AVE.
NEW ORLEANS, LA 70130

MY ROUTINE

NECESSARY COMPONENTS	PHASE I ___ - ___ WK	PHASE II ___ - ___ WK	MAINTENANCE
CARDIOVASCULAR FITNESS _____ X/WK	Target heart rate Blood Pressure Pulse	Target heart rate Blood Pressure Pulse	T. H. R. B. P. Pulse
MUSCULAR ST. & END _____ X/WK			
FLEXIBILITY _____ X/WK			
_____ X/WK			
_____ X/WK			

FITNESS LOG

YEAR _____   NAME _____

	1	2	3	4	5	6	7	8	9	10	11	12	13	14	15	16	17	18	19	20	21	22	23	24	25	26	27	28	29	30	31	TOTAL
JAN.																																
FEB.																																
MARCH																																
APRIL																																
MAY																																
JUNE																																
JULY																																
AUG.																																
SEPT.																																
OCT.																																
NOV.																																
DEC.																																

REMARKS: _____

179

"FEELING GREAT!" PROGRAM

NAME: _____   DATE: _____

GOALS: _____
_____
_____
_____
_____
_____

HOMEWORK: _____
_____
_____
_____
_____

PERIODIC REVIEW: _____
_____
_____
_____
_____
_____
_____
_____
_____
_____
_____

" Feeling Great!" Program
CONTRACT/GOALS FORM

Date: _____

I, _____ , hereby proclaim to work toward the following goals to the

best of my ability:

Long-range Goals:
(What improvements I want to accomplish six months from today)

1) _____

2) _____

3) _____

Short-range Goals:
(What I need to do now to reach my long-range goals)
(Excerise/Diet/Other)

1) _____

2) _____

3) _____

Signed_____

Witness_____

I understand that the fitness staff of the Lee Circle YMCA will be available for individual consultation
to help me pursue a healthier lifestyle.   My signature verifies my desire and commitment to accept the
challenge and self-responsibility of becoming a healthier individual.

2/88

" Feeling Great!"
PROGRAM EVALUATION

PROGRAM LEADER: _____ TODAY'S DATE: _____

COMMENTS ON PROGRAM:

	EXCELLENT	GOOD	FAIR	POOR
LEADERSHIP				
CLEANLINESS				
SAFETY				
PROGRAM CONTENT				
ORGANIZATION				
MET YOUR NEEDS				

PROGRAM STRENGTHS: _____

_____

PROGRAM WEAKNESSES: _____

_____

SUGGESTED IMPROVEMENTS: _____

_____

If you would like the program director to
contact you, please fill out below:

WE APPRECIATE YOUR COMMENTS!
Your evaluation and comments are important
as we work to maintain and improve our level
of quality and service to you.

NAME: _____

PHONE NUMBER: _____

" Feeling Great!" Program
RECOMMENDATIONS:

DATE: _____

I would like to suggest that:

_____

_____

_____

_____

_____

_____

_____

Please contact me regarding this matter at :
Phone Number _____

Name: _____

2/88

"FEELING GREAT!" DAILY ATTENDANCE

NAME — PHONE #	8/12	8/14	8/19	8/21	8/26	8/28	9/2	9/4	9/9	9/11	9/16	9/18	9/23	9/25	9/30	10/2	10/7	10/9	10/14	10/16	10/21
1.																					
2.																					
3.																					
4.																					
5.																					
6.																					
7.																					
8.																					
9.																					
10.																					
11.																					
12.																					
13.																					
14.																					
15.																					
16.																					
17.																					
18.																					
19.																					
20.																					
21.																					
22.																					
23.																					
24.																					
25.																					
26.																					
27.																					
28.																					
29.																					

"Feeling Great!" Program participant count and monies collected - Jules C. Weiss, M.A. ATR

January

of classes — 8
# of participants — 88
Average daily attendance — 11
# of members — 15
Monies collected — $131.00

February

of classes — 8
# of participants — 110
Average daily attendance — 14
# of members — 12
Monies collected — $210.50

March

of classes — 8
# of participants — 111
Average daily attendance — 14
# of members — 2
Monies collected — $249.25

April

of classes — 9
# of participants — 98
Average daily attendance — 11
# of members — 12
Monies collected — $158.00

May

of classes — 8
# of participants — 105
Average daily attendance — 13
# of members — 9
Monies collected — $221.25

June

of classes — 9
# of participants —113
Average daily attendance — 13
# of members — 13
Monies collected — $238.75

July

of classes — 7
# of participants — 103
Average daily attendance — 15
# of members — 6
Monies collected — $202.75

August

of classes — 8
# of participants — 117
Average daily attendance — 15
# of members — 7
Monies collected — $245.50

"Feeling Great!" Program participant count and monies collected - Jules C. Weiss, M.A. ATR

Date	Attendance	Members	Fees collected
8/12/86	18 people	(2 members)	$35.00
8/14/86	26 people	(2 members)	$59.75
8/19/86	24 people	(5 members)	$39.00
8/21/86	24 people	(3 members)	$53.00
8/26/86	16 people	(3 members)	$28.25
8/28/86	21 people	(3 members)	$45.25
9/2/86	19 people	(2 members)	$27.50
9/4/86	20 people	(3 members)	$43.00

165 - Total attendance
21 - av. per Tues & Thur
$330.75 fees collected
23 - members attended

Date	Attendance	Members	Fees collected
9/9/86	19 people	(3 members)	$40.00
9/11/86	28 people	(3 members)	$56.25
9/16/86	19 people	(3 members)	$35.50
9/18/86	18 people	(3 members)	$29.00
9/23/86	22 people	(3 members)	$44.00
9/25/86	24 people	(4 members)	$51.50
9/30/86	17 people	(3 members)	$25.00
10/2/86	19 people	(3 members)	$35.50

166 - Total attendance
21 - av. per Tues & Thur
$316.75 fees collected
25 - members attended

Date	Attendance	Members	Fees collected
10/7/86	20 people	(3 members)	$32.25
10/9/86	20 people	(3 members)	$38.75
10/14/86	21 people	(3 members)	$39.75
10/16/86	18 people	(3 members)	$30.75
10/21/86	17 people	(3 members)	$30.00
10/23/86	19 people	(3 members)	$39.75
10/28/86	15 people	(3 members)	$25.00
10/30/86	16 people	(2 members)	$29.00

146 - Total attendance
18 - av. per Tues & Thur
$265.25 fees collected
23 - members attended

Date	Attendance	Members	Fees collected
11/4/86	18 people	(3 members)	$30.75
11/6/86	17 people	(2 members)	$35.75
11/11/86	15 people	(3 members)	$23.25
11/13/86	14 people	(2 members)	$29.75
11/18/86	18 people	(3 members)	$29.00
11/20/86	20 people	(3 members)	$43.75
11/25/86	14 people	(2 members)	$30.50
11/27/86	Thanksgiving	Holiday	

116 - Total attendance
17 - av. per Tues & Thur
$222.75 fees collected
18 - members attended

WELCOME TO THE
"FEELING GREAT" PROGRAM

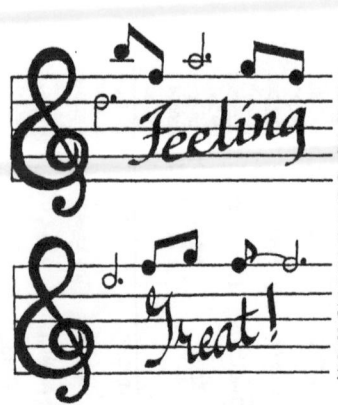

I am writing to acquaint participants and potential participants with the new exercise, swimming, and health education class at the Lee Circle YMCA, "FEELING GREAT!" program. This program is designed specifically for people over the age of fifty. It will be held on Tuesday and Thursday mornings from 9:00 - 11:30 and will include an exercise and relaxation session, a health-care lecture/discussion on topics pertinent to the older adult, and a swimming or active games session. Participants can take part in swimming lessons, water exercise or enjoy free time in the pool. Everyone is given a choice of participating in an active game or sport or going swimming. Following the morning program, an optional low-cost lunch is available at Back to the Garden restaurant at the YMCA. The cost of the program is $3.25 per day or $5.00 per week. With a month of regular attendance (of at least once a week) participants receive one free session.

Some of the questions you may have are listed below with an answer and explanation about the "FEELING GREAT!" program. If you have any other questions, feel free to call me, Jules Weiss, at 568-9622. If you can not reach me please leave a message and I will return your call as soon as possible. I look forward to seeing you at the "FEELING GREAT!" program.

1.   What should I wear or bring to wear?
     Participate can exercise in any loose fitting clothes but should bring something else to wear when they leave due to perspiration from exercising. If a participant chooses to swim, a bathing suit is mandatory. A locker room is provided for changing clothes before and after class. Participants can secure their clothes and personal possessions in a locker if they bring their own lock, or they may carry their clothes with them to the exercise room. For showering, participants need to bring their own shampoo. Sneakers are recommended for exercises and games.

2.   Can women come to the YMCA?
     Absolutely. Almost half of the members of the YMCA in New Orleans are women. The "FEELING GREAT!" program is designed for both men and women.

3.   If I am out of shape and rarely exercise, can I still participate?
     Yes! The classes are designed to slowly develop the important aspects of your physical fitness such as muscular endurance, muscle strength, joint flexibility, and cardiovascular conditioning. No one is too unfit for the program because each session is tailored to the participants' abilities and desires. In this program, it is not how good you look; it's how great you feel!

4.   If I currently exercise on a daily basis or weekly basis will the class be helpful?
     Yes! Participants will learn a range of exercises and new and varied ways to supplement their current programs. Emphasis will be placed on peer group activities for fun and enjoyment. In each session we will have a new health lecture and discussion, learning about staying well. Good health is not just exercising but is learning how to optimally take the best care of you body and maintain health and fitness awareness.

5. If I have arthritis can I participate?

Yes! Classes are specifically designed and tailored for people who have arthritis or similar problems. The classes covers a range of exercises which will benefit those suffering from arthritis pain and will provide exercises to do at home for continued improvement. It is a proven fact that water exercises are beneficial for persons with arthritis due to the fact that it takes the pressure off weight-bearing joints and allows a person to improve joint articulation without much of the discomfort which normally comes with movement.

6. If I have a heart condition can I participate?

Participants with a heart condition should talk to their doctor before beginning any exercise program. The YMCA strongly recommends that each participant have a doctor's permission to participate in an exercise program. In the "FEELING GREAT!" program, it is stressed that people do what they can, not to overwork themselves, but to go at their own pace. There is no pressure to perform in this program but a focus on Feeling Great!

7. If I have a handicap can I participate?

Yes! Everyone can participate to the best of his/her abilities. The program will have specifically designed activities for people of varying abilities and disabilities.

8. Do I have to go swimming if I participate in the "FEELING GREAT!" program?

No! Participants have a choice of either joining an active game or sport, continuing to exercise (use the jogging/walking track or other facilities), or going swimming.

9. How large will the class be?

Each class will have between five and twenty participants with one or two instructor.

10. Can I bring a guest?

Yes! We encourage participants to bring guests. We believe that "FEELING GREAT!" is a vital program for all senior adults. There will be no charge for the first class or if your guest just wants to watch.

11. Can I bring my own lunch to eat with my friends after class at Back to the Garden restaurant?

Yes! A major aspect of this program is having an enjoyable social time with your friends. Bring your lunch or buy it at the restaurant.

12. How much is lunch at Back to the Garden restaurant?

We will be having specially priced lunches for members of the "FEELING GREAT!" program. The cost will range from $1.50 to $3.00 per lunch with a variety of excellent food choices.

13. What facilities at the YMCA will be available to me during the "FEELING GREAT!" program?

Numerous YMCA facilities will be available to "FEELING GREAT!" program members such as the indoor gym, the indoor walking and jogging track, and indoor heated swimming pool, an exercise and activity room, and a complete dressing, shower, and locker room facilities for men and women.

14. When can I join?

Participants can join at any time. The "FEELING GREAT!" program provides ongoing sessions in exercise, activities, swimming, and fitness, with different lectures and discussions on health related topics in each class.

15. When do I pay for the class?

Participants can pay at 9:00 AM (at the Control Point at the YMCA before class) for that day or for future classes. Participants will receive a monthly card to designate that they are in the "FEELING GREAT!" program and a cash receipt for payment of classes.

16. Where does the class meet?

    Participants will pay for the class and gather at the control point-front desk at the Lee Circle YMCA at 9:00 AM on Tuesday and Thursday mornings.

17. Can anyone help me get to the bus after the program?

    Yes! The YMCA staff or Lee Circle front desk guard will be happy to escort you to the bus or the St. Charles Streetcar.

18. How can I get to the program?

    The program is located at the Lee Circle YMCA in downtown New Orleans. For people who do not have a car, the St. Charles Streetcar stops at Lee Circle right next to the YMCA. The Freret, Magazine, and Jackson buses stop within walking distance of the Lee Circle YMCA. Another option is to take any other bus to Canal Street and transfer to the St. Charles Streetcar. Some senior citizen centers and facilities will be using their own vans to transport participants. Street and lot parking is available adjacent to the YMCA entrance.

19. Are there any other "FEELING GREAT!" programs in the city?

    No, not at this time; but in the near future we hope to start "FEELING GREAT!" programs at branch YMCA's throughout the metropolitan New Orleans area.

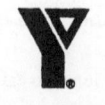

Lee Circle YMCA
936 St. Charles Avenue
New Orleans, LA 70130
(504) 568-9622

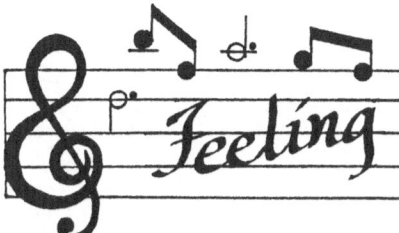

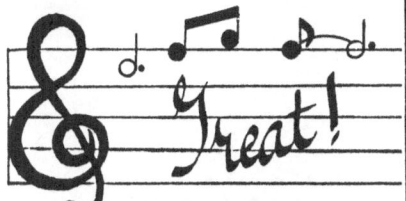

**A new program
from the YMCA
for men and women
over the age of 50!**

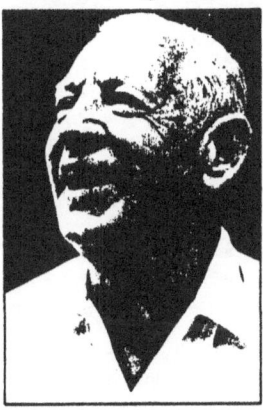

Feeling Great! Coordinators

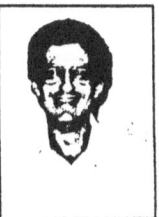

Jules C. Weiss

Jules C. Weiss, M.A., is a Registered Art Therapist who has worked as a counselor and program coordinator for adults for over ten years. He holds a Masters Degree in Creative Arts Therapy, is trained in counseling and art, music, and movement therapy, and recently completed a book on his work, **Expressive Therapy With Elders And The Disabled: Touching The Heart of Life.**

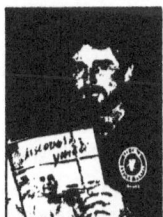

Howard Leighton

Howard Leighton, Health and Fitness Director of the Lee Circle YMCA, has been involved with adult fitness programs for the last 10 years. Howard is Director of the Human Performance lab at the Lee Circle YMCA and is a certified instructor through the YMCA in the "Y's Way to a Healthy Back" and "Y's Way to Physical Fitness."

For more information, call 568-9622.

The YMCA believes that total health is part of a life-long venture. **Feeling Great!**, an exercise, swimming, and health program, was created for adults over 50 who wish to maintain their physical well-being through exercise, health education, activity, and having fun.

Feeling Great! includes the following components:

* Exercise and relaxation class
* Home health and fitness tips
* Lectures and discussions on health care issues and preventive medicine
* Optional swimming lessons and water exercise
* Optional free time in the pool for fun
* Health assessment and monitoring
* Games and sports with your friends
* Use of exercise equipment and facilities at the Lee Circle YMCA
* An optional, low-cost, nutritious lunch at the Back to the Garden Restaurant at the YMCA.

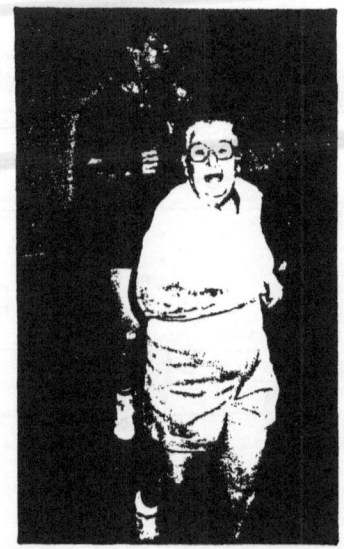

PARTICIPANTS RESPOND

"After 3 weeks in the program I can walk up and down stairs, where before I couldn't do that without terrible pain."
—Mary C. age 70+

"I'm not as tired as before and I feel better about myself."
—Delores J. age 51

"I was recovering from a stroke when I joined. It has really helped my whole life. I've improved my range of motion, leg strength, and arm and hand strength."
—Marie T. age 70

Feeling Great! will be offered from 9:00-11:30 AM every Tuesday and Thursday at the Lee Circle YMCA.

45 minutes—Exercise and Relaxation
30 minutes—Health Care lectures/discussions
45 minutes—Choice of swimming, active games, sports, exercises, or walking/jogging
Plus—time for an optional lunch with your friends.

COST: $3.25 per session or $5.00 per week (Lunch is extra).

Group Rates available.

SPECIAL OFFER

For every month of regular attendance (of at least once a week), you'll receive ONE FREE SESSION!

SAMPLE TOPICS FOR
HEALTH LECTURES/DISCUSSIONS

* Stress Management/Relaxation
* Exercise for the older adult
* The Y's way to a healthy back
* Nutrition/Diet
* Healthy lifestyles
* Alleviating high blood pressure
* Resources in the city for exercise, enjoyment, entertainment, and learning
* And many more!

YOU ARE INVITED to participate. Plan to join us at 9:00 AM on Tuesdays and Thursdays at the Lee Circle YMCA, 936 St. Charles Avenue. You can join at anytime for one or two days a week. Pay as you go.

Just send in the attached registration card or call us at 568-9622 to reserve your place.

Transportation to Lee Circle:
1. The St. Charles Streetcar stops at Lee Circle right next to the YMCA.
2. The Freret, Magazine, and Jackson buses stop within walking distance of the Lee Circle YMCA.
3. Take any other bus to Canal Street and transfer to the St. Charles Streetcar.
4. If you drive, parking is available at the Lee Circle Texaco station for $2.00.
5. For Van transportation (pick-up at your home), call Allegra "Rose" Matthews at 486-5177 or 891-2457.

REGISTRATION

NAME: _____

ADDRESS: _____
(Street No. and/or Apt. No.)

_____
(City)   (State)   (Zip)

PHONE: _____

EMERGENCY CONTACT:

_____
(Name)

_____
(Phone)

Activity Level (Circle One):

High   Low

Day(s) you'll probably participate (Circle one or both):

Tuesday   Thursday

I understand that the YMCA strongly recommends that each participant have a doctor's permission to participate in an exercise program. My signature on this form indicates my willingness to accept complete responsibility for my physical well-being. The YMCA is hereby relieved of all responsibility or liability associated with my participation in the **Feeling Great!** program.

_____   _____
Signature   Date

Chapter VII

Conclusion

This book is a reflection of a vital program that addresses the health care needs and concerns of older adults. It describes an exercise program that helps people, many who have not exercised in years, to once again regain or continue to develop the strength, vitality, and beauty of their body, mind, and spirit.

Good health care for older adults is everyone's concern; for if we have our health we will all become senior citizens someday. Due to the advances in medical technology and other positive life factors, there is a tremendous growth in the older adult population. Currently one out of nine people are over 65. In less than fifty years, by the year 2030, it is predicted that one out of five people will be over 65. The fastest growing segment of our population is those who are 85 and older. The growth of the 85 + population raises the concern for quality long-term care and residential facilities which are both medically equipped and emotionally satisfying for the lifelong growth and happiness of senior citizens.

There is a great need among older adults to learn and practice preventive health care and to discover ways to enrich and live fulfilling lives. The body will naturally age, but how it ages is our choice. If senior citizens give up in a state of depression or apathy, and neglect the health of their body, mind and spirit, they will eventually weaken physically and become susceptible to sickness, ill-health, and physical and emotional discomfort. With a good attitude, a healthy environment, peer support, and a commitment to their well-being, the mind and spirit can stay invigorated and vital. This type of attitude can motivate individuals to continue to grow and develop through their daily activities, social life, and personal wellness program.

PROBLEMS/SOLUTIONS

Emotional Needs

Depression is the number one mental health problem for older adults. This problem reflects feelings of limited options and resources which is encumbered by the possible accompanying grief over not possessing the health, vitality, and opportunities of their youth. Often depression is anger focused inwardly. Anger due to the limitations and road blocks in a person's life needs to be addressed and properly dealt with before it festers and causes further emotional and possible physical harm. Peer support and opportunities for emotional, physical, and psychological growth and satisfaction may be the number one solution for depression.

When the body becomes ill, a doctor can give medications to help the cause and symptoms of the illness. But, when the mind becomes desperate, depressed, or mentally ill, medications may offer only temporary relief, and other resources are needed such as peer support and motivation. Often, mental problems can create additional physical illnesses through stress and tension. Some of the stressful issues facing senior citizens are: worry over paying for medical bills on a limited budget, the depressing thoughts of possibly not regaining their health, changes in lifestyle and options due to illness and loss, and other related issues. Without motivation, desire, hope, and fulfilling opportunities, depression can set in and crumble the very existence of a person.

Many older adults do not feel in control of their lives as they were when they were younger. They may be retired and living in a different home situation with limited financial resources, social networking and opportunities. Lack of independence is a major issue and problem for many older adults. This is one reason why senior citizens so desperately need good supportive programs that encourage and assist them with independent living and meet their crucial psychosocial needs in a mature manner.

Many people with chronic illnesses or problems, or who are in stressful situations feel isolated and alone without a supportive person or group to discuss their situation with. This form of isolation can be traumatic and cause feelings of anger, unjustness, discontentment, and possibly a feeling of spiritual emptiness and bitterness toward a person's faith/religion.

Support groups which focus on problems, needs, similar concerns, and peer guidance can help people from disengaging and becoming socially isolated. Through sharing concerns and receiving feedback and support, these groups can offer meaningful dialogue, a sense of security, intimacy, nurturance, along with a feeling of belonging and approval. Support groups are a lifeline to many people who are troubled by everyday problems. An exercise/health education program, like the "Feeling Great!" program, can be an opportunity for a support group.

Physical Needs

Exercise and health education is everyone's concern. Dr. Warshaw writes in his book *Managing Stress*:

> Its exact incidence is not known, but it has been said that 80 percent of the population will experience at least one disabling episode during adult life. Most backaches are attributed to an acute strain or trauma resulting from an attempt to lift something or an injudicious movement. Careful investigation, however, frequently reveals that the precipitating incident was co-incidental, the real cause being chronic tension, stiffness, and weakness of key postural muscles induced by stress. Especially in sedentary individuals in whom these muscles are weakened by inactivity, the tension itself can produce a soreness but, more important, it also leaves the muscles vulnerable to injury by a sudden or strenuous movement.

Sedentary older adults are more vulnerable to injuries due to their physical condition. This is complicated by the aging of the body which, in case of injury, causes the healing process to take longer.

Arthritis is the number one physical problem of older adults and besides aspirin, exercise is one of the primary remedies for relief and physical improvement. Exercise programs for older adults are too few and far between to meet the great need of older adults in this country today. There are many commercials that advertise medications for people suffering from arthritis pain. But, it is rare to ever see an exercise program advertised for arthritis sufferers which in the long run may provide many older adults with more long-term relief.

Most senior citizens are very concerned about their health and are willing to do what it takes to become healthier. If this is true why is it so common to hear that many elderly people are being misdiagnosed, overmedicated, and suffer from poor health? Why is the highest number of suicides occurring in the segment of our population who are age 75 and older? Of course it is true that the normal aging of the body can bring about new problems and concerns. But this problem is tremendously compounded by the lack in our current health care system to sufficiently address the long-term physical needs of older adults. There is a lack of resources in preventive health care, supportive programs for all older adults with varying medical, social and psychological needs, and networking between federal, state, city, and private health care organizations. These services need to reach the public and meet the overwhelming health cry of older adults desiring good health care which everyone deserves. But unfortunately, there are various missing links in our health care system.

One link is in the poor dissemination of health care information and another in the lack of exercise/health education/peer support programs that meet the vital needs of various ethnic and/or social, senior citizen groups. There is an abundance of good health care information that many governmental agencies and other organizations already possess and distribute on a limited basis to some groups and also offer upon request to the general public. But, often the public does not know what materials are available and where to write for the information.

Health care information needs to be systematically disseminated to all senior citizens. Similar to receiving their social security checks, they should also receive health care bulletins on the latest research, programs, and products for older adults. Initiating and distributing nationwide preventive health care bulletins along with conducting exercise/health education/peer support programs throughout the country could save millions of dollars in health care costs. Along with the savings in health care costs, it would greatly aid the older adult population in being more knowledgeable about aging and what is needed to stay healthy. Finally as a result of a nation-wide health program it may motivate people to become more in-volved with taking responsibility for their health, develop commu-nity support and programs, and enhance their lives.

Quality exercise/health education/peer support programs are im-perative for the well-being of older adults. Programs should be held everywhere older adults congregate such as senior citizen centers, adult day care centers, at continuing education programs in colleges and high schools, at V.F.W. posts, and at hospitals and clinics. Everyone who gets a social security card should be offered the op-portunity to take an exercise/health education/aging class to learn how to master their life in the midst of physical, psychological, and social changes.

Growing old has many challenges. But it gets even harder when the individual does not have the essential tools such as knowledge of exercise, proper nutrition, peer support, the understanding of the changes in the body due to aging along with the needed attention to certain medical tests. For older adults, understanding the complex-ity and ingredients for optimal psycho-social-physical well-being is essential, especially in the modern day maze of health care services and products.

UNIVERSITIES FOR
GROWING OLDER/GROWING YOUNGER

Universities and schools need to offer quality programs for older adults which are invigorating. They need to help people who are making major life transitions and offer special educational, crea-tive, and coping skills. A few of the many courses which should be taught are: retirement and entering new professions; dealing with issues of loss, grief, and loneliness; learning about nutrition, exer-cise, preventive medicine, and wholistic health care; social net-working — adjusting to new roles and creating new roles in life; lei-sure and creative activities.

These schools are not a frill in life but rather a necessity. Similar to the necessity of public education for the growing child to learn, adjust, and find his/her place in society, it is vital to have programs for older adults that addresses their educational, social, psychological and physical needs and desires. Life changes do not have to be crises, but rather can be exciting transitions to new learning, experiences, and relationships. Older adults can feel renewed with the help of a supportive program to learn and share with others. This must also be supported by a community that cares and respects the needs and talents of older adults. Universities for older adults need to help inspire, motivate, and teach people the desired skills to aid them in growing older with dignity, self-respect, and a vitality for life. Our greatest untapped resource may be the older adult generation.

To empower senior citizens to take charge of their life, become wise consumers, understand the health care system, the politics of government and their community will make them more effective leaders of their generation. Senior citizens can help to bridge the gap between various segments of the community. There is no greater teacher than experience and senior citizens have a corner on the experiential market. So let the wise elder be recognized, let the years be shared, and let the wisdom of the ages be among us. Allow the older adult to be a respected, valuable nurturer and teacher in our community. And, may the government, various professional organizations, universities and colleges help senior citizens by sharing with them the newest technology health care to assist in staying healthy and vibrant in the "face" of aging; to feel ageless.

AGELESS AGING

Many times I have asked active older adults, ages 60 to 100, how old do they feel. They responded by saying something which surprised me. They did not feel any age at all. They just felt comfortable with themselves. This seemed to be agelessly aging — living with integrity, respect, and an understanding of the stages of their lives.

There may be no conclusion to life, only being and growing. As we grow we change; even death is just a change in the physical property of the self, the soul lives on. The time we spend keeping our body and mind in shape reflects the testimony of our life, the refinement of our soul, to be tools in the light of grace. The grace that brought us to life and the same grace that takes us from this world.

We are given one life to grow, learn, love and be loved. We are also given the responsibility to take care of the gift of life, ours and others. Let us respect the honor bestowed upon us and thank God for the opportunity to live a healthy life. Let us be dedicated, committed to the health of the world.

> The sage asks the student
> "What is the moment to live for?"
> The student replies,
> "To listen to the bells."
> The sage agrees and comments,
> "When you hear the bells
> the sound becomes a part of you.
> Similar to hearing the teachings of wisdom,
> you become the teachings and forthright the teacher.
> Every student is a teacher
> and every teacher a student."